Kama Su

2 Books in

Kama Sutra for Beginners and Sex Positions. The MOST Practical Guide with 150+ POSITIONS for Couples with Advanced Techniques to Make WILD SEX and EXPLODE your Private Life.

Lana Fox

Kama Sutra for Beginners

A Practical Guide on KAMA SUTRA with Various SEX POSITIONS for Couples to Make WILD SEX with SECRET Strategies for Men and Women (Before and During Foreplay)

Lana Fox

Table of Contents

Introduction 9

Chapter 1: Communication 13

Chapter 2: Before and during Foreplay 29

Chapter 3: Sex.. 67

Chapter 4: Making Yourself Attractive 84

Chapter 5: Keep It Up... 97

Conclusion 103

Introduction

Congratulations on purchasing this book and thank you for doing so. There are plenty of books on this subject out there on the market, but you chose this one and it is much appreciated that you did so!

The ensuing chapters will discuss a variety of topics, including physical intimacy, flirtation, foreplay, and communication between sexual partners. The key to understanding and getting the full gist of what this eBook is about is to simply use it as a sort of stepping stone, the first step in getting to know what the actual Kama Sutra is really about. True, the ancient Hindu text does indeed discuss sexual positions, techniques, and practices at length. After all, it is the most well-known aspect of the book. But, believe it or not, a greater portion of the book also speaks in depth about searching out a life partner or spouse, improving your personal physical attractiveness (which will also be discussed in this eBook), improving your station in life, and the attainment of being a true, faithful, and virtuous person. Obviously, physical intimacy is absolutely a key element in enhancing the sex life of a couple, but attention to one's personal wishes, needs, desires, and listening to what your partner wants on a physical and emotional level, and taking the needed steps to ensure these goals are met are also equally as important.

Remember, the word kama (meaning desire) is drawn from one of the four goals of Hindu existence, (the others being artha, which is material prosperity, dharma, which is living a virtuous life, and moksha, which means liberation). Sutra simply means rules or things that hold the concept together and acts as a tying bind. In other words, Kama Sutra, roughly translated, is the rules of desire to enhance your overall life and existence! Taking a cue from this, a couple just starting out in a relationship, or having been in an intimate relationship for quite a while, can discover certain techniques (physical and otherwise) that will add a spark of sensuality to their relationship, and find ways and means that will allow that one single spark to ignite and spread a great and glorious fire between the two of them. And as the ancient Hindu texts, the Vedas, tell us, the universe was created by a massive, wonderful heat and soon after, desire followed.

Again, we can't thank you enough for deciding to purchase this book. Every possible effort was made to ensure that it is full of as much useful information as possible, and the explanations, steps, and advice are written in a way that can be clearly understood. All couples, whether they are straight, gay, Bi, trans, in a monogamous relationship, open relationship, or whatever the case, old, young, middle-aged, or otherwise, deserve to be happy and to feel fulfilled on all levels, physically, mentally, spiritually, and emotionally. This is the primary aim of this text. Please enjoy, and if you like what you read here, please recommend it to others as well!

Before you begin, you should know that this book is not about how you can be a sex god in the bedroom. It is about being an attentive lover and devoting yourself to the pleasure of your partner. Doing so will bring you higher pleasure as well.

If you are looking to create a more intimate environment for you and your partner, this is a great book to instruct you on how to do so.

Enjoy this book, and enjoy spicing up your life in and outside of the bedroom.

Chapter 1: Communication

Yes. It's true. The Kama Sutra is filled with vivid descriptions and illustrations of two people in a variety of sexual positions. Some positions are, let's face it, relatively standard that we all know, or have seen, or have heard about, or have tried, or just know how to do instinctively. And other positions look like anyone over the age of 40 will run the risk of dislocating a hip or, at the very least, throw their back out if they try them! And there are even a few positions that require a person to be a gymnast or contortionist to even get close to getting right! One look at some of the drawings in that ancient text might have one reaching for a magnifying glass for a closer look to see if they're actually seeing what they're seeing.

A lot of people have heard the term. (Often mispronounced as Karma Sutra) However, not a lot of people really can define the term as a whole. They know that it relates to sex, but they are not sure exactly what it is that the term implies.

Well, you are right that it relates to sex, but that is not really the entire truth. Kamasutra is a type of romancing and getting intimate with your partner that reaches a realm completely outside of sex to make sex more interesting and more intense.

While the term relies heavily on sexual positions in today's age, it still revolves around the idea that humans are inherently sexual creatures, and to staunch that sexuality is inhumane and cruel to our bodies. It brings sex out of the bedroom, and into the rest of the world in a way that makes it feel discreet and yet oh so naughty at the same time.

If you are a shy person and feel that you would not be able to do anything sexual in public, do not worry. You are most likely not going to go for a quick shag in the park. (Unless that is something you are into, though you could run into some serious legal issues if you are caught) Most of the sexuality out in your public life relies on gestures and body language, minute and subtle touches, and communication to drive the mind wild. You could be preparing your partner for the bedroom, and the people around you could have no idea what you are doing, or that you are even doing anything. That is the wonderful thing about Kamasutra. You can do all the dirty things you could imagine, and no one else than your partner would be the wiser.

But, as stated in the introduction to this eBook, the physical side of a sexual relationship is only one part of intimacy. Vātsyāyana, the Indian philosopher who scribed the Kama Sutra, understood that to attain a healthy, open, and fulfilled sexual relationship, a person has to feel fulfilled, or strive to feel fulfilled, on all levels (in their home, in their working life, and in life in general). And even though the physical part of the Kama Sutra is what it's known for, Vātsyāyana spends maybe a quarter or a third (depending on the translated copy that you read) of the text describing sex positions. The majority focuses on other aspects of a couple's personal relationship, and how a person can move towards fulfillment.

But how do we get there? How do we begin moving closer to a well-rounded, complete sex life with our partners?

The answer is communication.

Talking

Although admittedly, starting off any text with paragraphs about talking isn't as enticing or sexy as advice on oral sex, mutual masturbation, or intercourse, there's a simple reason why we chose to place the aspects of communication as the very first chapter in this book. You can't be satisfied in a sexual relationship with your partner unless you can actually tell them exactly what it is that you want! And, on the flip side, you can't complete your partner's wishes unless they tell you who they really are and what they want. The communication factor between any couple at any level of their relationship, whether it's in the initial stages or many years on, has to be a top priority, and must continue to be a top priority for the absolute duration of the relationship.

Consider this scenario, if you will. A wife who's been married to her husband for a couple of years, has, for many years up until that point, wanted to experience a three-way with her husband and another man. She's thought about it numerous times, fantasized about it in her alone time, dreamed about it, and craved it. However, she's never brought it up to him. It wasn't because of anything that he's ever said or done. He's not a prude, and he's not closed-minded when it comes to the bedroom. Perhaps it's because of social conditioning ("A good wife would never do something so slutty!"), or she may be fearful of the answer he may give. Maybe the thought of another man in the bedroom with them might make him feel threatened. Whatever the case is, unless she feels comfortable enough to bring this to the attention of her husband, she may feel empty, or, at the very least, unfulfilled sexually. No one should ever have to feel that way.

Here's another one. Let's say a husband wants to share his interest in role-playing in the bedroom with his wife. He has this fantasy about being the boss of a big company, and he wants his "secretary" (his wife) to stay after work on that day to *ahem* get to know her better. But his wife has never given the signal in the time that they've known each other that she would be into such things. Should he bring it up? Should he just keep his mouth shut? Or will he just ignore that desire and move on?

In either case of the wife or the husband, keeping what you want completely emerged beneath the surface of yourself does NOT get rid of the desire at all. It always will be there. And, unfortunately, as time goes on, the longer that something lies under the surface, five possible outcomes could occur:

• It's never fully realized or tried, and therefore the person doesn't feel complete when it comes to satisfying their sexual desires.

17

•   A person craves this desire so deeply and absolutely doesn't feel that they can bring about a conversation addressing this desire to their spouse or significant other, and thus they seek out another person to fulfill this desire, which, obviously, leads to cheating, adultery, dishonesty, etc.

•   It's brought to the surface, it's communicated clearly, and the partner soundly rejects it, which may lead to either outcome previously discussed in one or two.

•   It's brought to the surface, it's communicated clearly, and the partner rejects it in a kind, understanding manner, stating that the kink, fetish, interest, or whatever it is, may not interest them. But, they're willing to try something similar, etc., and satisfaction can be attained in this exploration, or, at least, the avenues of communication have been opened on the subject.

•   Or it's brought to the surface, communicated, shared, the partner agrees, and the interest or desire has been achieved.

It may sound cliché, and it may go without saying, but communication is a two-way street. You have an idea, you have a goal, and you have something that you want to try. Therefore, you need to communicate it in a logical, clear, and respectful manner. In other words, you have to adhere to the supreme, top, prime, absolute, number one rule in effective communication: Know your audience and know how to talk to them. If your partner needs things explained in full detail, then full detail is what you should give. If your partner is more receptive to talking over dinner or drinks, then go with that. You need to do everything you can to communicate efficiently and clearly.

But you have to go into the scenario, from the outset, with the complete understanding that the person you're communicating your message to may or may not accept it, especially if your kink, fetish, or tend to run on the darker side of things. If you've wanted to try water sports' (also commonly referred to as 'golden showers,' or 'piss play') and your partner certainly does not want to do this in the slightest, you have to keep in mind that this desire might never come to fruition between you and your significant other. You have to get your needs and wants out there, but, on the other side of the coin, you have to understand their needs and wants as well.

Again, it's a two-way street.

Listening

And going to the other side of that two-way street…

You as a partner in an intimate relationship need to be empathetic to the person communicating their message to you. Just because you may not like the idea of, say, pegging or anal sex or whatever, it doesn't mean you should automatically put restrictions on it. Always keep an open mind. Hear what your spouse, boyfriend, or girlfriend, has to say. And keep in mind one crucial thing, a person needs, wants and deserves to feel complete physically, mentally, emotionally, and spiritually in a relationship. Helping them achieve this will only draw two people closer, and the level of depth of their relationship will become greater. As Vātsyāyana himself said in the closing of the Kama Sutra, "A person… who preserves his Dharma, his Artha, and his Kama, and who has regard to the customs, is sure to obtain the mastery over his senses. In short, an intelligent and knowing person attending to Dharma and Artha and also to the Kama, without becoming the slave of his passions, will obtain success."

After your partner has shared their desires with you, faithful consideration must be given to the idea, and a logical, understanding answer must be given. Not to sound like a broken record, but empathy is key. If you communicated something that you needed from another person, you do not want to hear an answer that falls along the lines of "I'll get back with you," or "I'll take that into consideration" or something that is sort of a verbal blow-off. You would be rather upset or disappointed, wouldn't you? Your partner took the time, effort, and guts to get that message to you. Essentially, they are saying (without actually coming out and saying it) that they want you — yes, you — above everyone else on planet Earth to help them achieve their sexual goals and realize their lusts, kinks, or desires. You! Not the neighbor. Not the co-worker. Not the celebrity they have in their personal fantasies. You. On that merit alone, a person deserves a thoughtful, grateful response.

What to Say, How to Say It, and When to Say It

If you were in the middle of fixing your car, and your wife began talking to you about fixing the gutters, you might get a little annoyed. If you have just gotten home from work, had a horrible day, are completely tired and just need to sit and relax for a moment, and your husband comes over to you and complains that you left the garage door open all day and that you need to stop being so forgetful, again, you'd be pretty irritated and it would probably result in a huge argument. Simply put, you don't just pay attention to the person you're trying to communicate with, but you also have to take into account the circumstances that the person is in, or the day they've had, and how they're responding to both. Pick your spots carefully. Choose your moment. Know what, how, and when to speak your message and when you want to convey that message.

And speaking of the 'when' aspect of the situation, if you can't have the conversation at a certain point throughout the day, but you want to have it soon, you need to know how to communicate that as well. If you send a text to your partner during the workday that says something along the lines of, "We need to talk, ASAP," they're probably going to think that something is seriously wrong, or that the conversation will be a very heated one. It also might not be a good idea to tell your partner just before they're leaving for work or for a day out with their friends that when they get back, "You and I need to have a discussion." Again, this will probably put the person on the defensive, or make them overly concerned, or have their minds dwell on something all day. Avoid saying something like this at all costs. Always keep in mind another strong tenant of communication, it's not how you 'say' something, it's 'how' you say something.

Whatever you need to do to gently, easily, logically, and, most of all, empathetically get across that you'd like to have a conversation with your loved one, do it. Don't make it seem like a life or death matter. Don't make it seem like you're about to lawyer-up and get those divorce papers in order. Make it seem like what you two need to discuss is important, but can wait until both of you are ready to sit down, happy, content, and open to one another.

When considering the moment when two people actually find the moment and the time in the day to talk, the two of them have to wait for a quiet moment when they can focus one hundred percent of their attention on one another. In this modern day, technologically enhanced, plugged in, selfie-taking, status updated, constantly conveyed the world that we live in, this is probably one of the hardest things that two people (especially younger people) will have to do. But it needs to be done.

Wait until all distractions are removed from your personal space, and the number one distraction in this day and age is the cell phone. Do not look at your cell phone when you are about to have a conversation with your partner. Don't! Avoid it entirely! Stop it now! Do not hold it. Do not cradle it. Put the phone away, do not answer it, do not respond to texts, do not check your apps, do not check status updates on Twitter or Facebook, do not FaceTime, do not do anything, anything at all, with your phone. Put it in the other room if you have to. Leave it out in the car. Have your partner hide it somewhere for the time being. Do anything you can to get the damn thing away from you!

For people who rely on their phone for their business, or for people who have basically grown up with a cell phone grafted to their hand since the age of five, the very idea of putting a phone away, or shutting it off, or not having the chance to look at it for an extended period of time can be scary. What if my client needs to get ahold of me? What if my boss sends me a text and needs to discuss something? What if my sister has her baby? What if my mom posts a new picture from her vacation? These are things that can wait. They have to. If you're the phone-addicted one in the relationship, and your partner said that they need to speak to you, you have to get it in your head that your loved one needs to talk to you about a serious matter without you being easily distracted like a dog that saw a squirrel run across the lawn. If you're the one that needs to say something, don't pause every five seconds during the communication of your 'serious' issue to pick up your phone and have a chat with some random person while your significant other sits there and waits and twiddles their thumbs until you're finished. It's not fair to them, it's not courteous, and, frankly, they won't take what you have to say seriously, because, obviously, you're not taking what you have to say seriously.

So, it cannot be stressed enough, get rid of the phone.

In addition to the cellphone, please, please, please shut off your tablet or laptop as well (you don't want email after email popping up during the conversation, or someone requesting a Skype, or an IM going off every few seconds), turn off the TV (who really cares who wins on Family Feud that evening?), shut off the radio (you've heard that Led Zeppelin or that Marvin Gaye or that Adele song hundreds of times before), close the door, sit in a chair, lay on the bed, or just stand there and look at and listen to one another.

Also, keep in mind that it might be best to avoid having the conversation just before bedtime in case the conversation runs a little long. And it might be best to avoid having it first thing in the morning. You need to have a clear head when conveying a message and when you're receiving a message. Tiredness plays havoc on your mind, and you don't need that. Find a time, any time that will do, during the day to be alone, focused, and open with one another.

And then...just talk. As stated, explain what you want sexually. Don't feel inhibited. Don't hold anything back. Open up. Be honest here. It's hard, it's difficult, yes, but you need to do it. Sharing details about what you want, even if it's with someone you love and care for, is never easy. Perhaps it's, again, social conditioning. In many areas of this world, talking about sex, sexuality, sexual activity, and wants, needs, kinks, and the like is considered taboo in so-called polite society. But we have to get past that. For two people to have a lasting, loving, wonderful relationship, honesty both in communication and in action is the prime element.

And, if you're the one hearing your partner, you also need to listen to them. That sounds like a redundancy, right? Hearing is listening, correct? But it really isn't. Hearing is automatic. Listening is an active thing. You hear sounds all around you at all times. However, are you listening? Are you consciously taking them in?

Listening means you have to willfully engage yourself. You have to tell yourself that you will receive whatever the message is and take it in, consider it, reflect on it, and give a response. And not only do we have to listen, but we also have to listen without any sort of prejudice or preconceived notions. This person whom you love and cherish has a very important message they want to share, and it's your responsibility to listen, consider, and respond to them.

Finally

Let's say you've had the conversation and everything went well. Perfect! Now you just have to find the time to take what you'd like to do to go to the next level.

But if the conversation didn't go all that great? Well, you just have to regroup. Maybe you weren't clear enough with your message. Maybe your partner was distracted. It's okay. Don't think about of giving up. Things like that happen from time to time in a relationship. But if you love your partner and have a deep respect for them, you'll do your best to communicate with them or find better ways to communicate with them or find better ways to receive their communications.

The trick here, people, is to not just come up with a plan of talking and emoting and conveying ideas and feelings. It's to keep it going, on and on throughout the years. As stated, clear communication should be the top priority in your relationship over the duration of it. Communication leads to deeper love and understanding, and if two things in this world are worth doing almost anything for, they are love and understanding.
And to quote the *Kama Sutra*, "A person who does, nothing will enjoy no happiness."

Chapter 2: Before and during Foreplay

Start out Slow

Okay, now here is some real talk. Foreplay still exists, people! Anymore, it seems like sex has no beginning, you just jump right in and go for two to five minutes, and then you are done. No wonder sex does not seem satisfying to a lot of couples. You have to warm up first. You don't run a marathon without stretching first, so why would you have sex without warming up the goods?

Foreplay also helps you avoid injury and after sex discomfort, because both people involved will be ready to go, rather than one partner being completely ready, and the other one not quite. Women especially need to be warmed up so that they can be properly lubricated to avoid unwanted friction rashes and possible vaginal tearing. Of course, those are worst case scenarios, but it is still possible and should be avoided at all costs.

For those of you rolling your eyes at the thought of foreplay, obviously, you have not experienced the right kind. It is not just oral and playing with each other's genitals. In fact, it is quite the opposite. Foreplay should involve minimal touching of the genital areas in the beginning. There are so many other ways to get in the mood other than what you would think is considered foreplay. Foreplay can start from the moment you wake up, and not end until the evening when you and your partner finally slip away into the bliss that is intense love making.

Mental Foreplay

It is no secret that the mind is the greatest sexual organ there is. You could have all of the stimulation in the world, but if the mind is not in it, then you will find that you have a really tough time experiencing any pleasure, let alone achieving an orgasm. So including the mind is an important thing to do for both you and your partner. You have to make sure that you are stimulating the mind properly though. You can't just say "Wanna have sex?" and leave it at that. You have to make your partner, and yourself, wild with desire at the thought of making love.

There are several ways to go about this. However, the easiest way to do so is to ease into it, starting in the morning. Wake your partner up with a slow, sensual kiss and tell them that you wish it was already the evening. As they get dressed, watch them, and undress them with your eyes. Make sure they notice you watching. Caress their back, and kiss them as you both part ways for the work day. By that time, both of you should be reeling with anticipation for the work day to be over. However, you should not stop there.

If you are allowed to have your phone at work, and your partner is as well, even just on your breaks, text them. Not just normal daily texts though. Make it sensual. "I can't wait to get you home" is just enough of a tease to make your partner excited for the night to come. If you have the time, try a little sexting if you feel up to it. You can tell your partner all the things that you would like to do to them, and get yourself, and your partner going, before you even get home.

There are so many ways you can mentally stimulate your partner. It goes hand in hand with getting them to relax as well, which was mentioned in a previous chapter.

Physical Foreplay

This is something that a lot of people think of when they think of foreplay. However, they think the genital aspect of it. There is so much more to even physical foreplay than a lot of people realize. You have to stimulate the entire body, not just the genitals. Even though they are the main contender in sex, the genitals are actually the least important part of foreplay. You have to focus on the other erogenous zones. The body has a lot of them.

A lot of people know that the neck tends to be one of them, and you can't deny that there is nothing more craze-inducing than a well-placed neck kiss or bite, but did you know that the earlobe is just as sensitive, if not more than the neck? They eyelids are actually very sensitive as well. Have your partner close their eyes, and gently trace the shape of their eyelids and watch them shudder in delight.

You also don't have to do physical foreplay in just the bedroom either. You can do physical foreplay wherever you are. For example, in the grocery store, you can come up behind you partner and run your hands down their arms while placing a gentle kiss on the back of their neck. You can do foreplay at home while watching a movie, by kissing various parts of your lover's body as they are distracted and turned away from you.

Showering or Bathing Together

This is something that a lot of couples today view as unnecessary. In fact, some people consider it as one person getting the steamy water, and one person in the cold corner the entire time. However, if done correctly, bathing or showering together could be very stimulating to both partners.

To do this efficiently, both partners must be able to enjoy the steamy hot water on their skin. Press your bodies together under the water as you kiss, and you will find that the water makes everything that much more stimulating. Stroke your partner's body with your hands, and kiss their neck. Groom them, and allow them to groom you. Whether it be with shaving, shampooing or soaping the body, they all can be sensual and intense sensations when combined with the steam and heat of the water on your skin. This is a type of foreplay that almost always leads to sex, so be sure to take your time and really focus on stimulating your partner.

Massage

This is another part of being intimate that is sorely overlooked. A massage can be a great way to help your partner relax after a long day and can be a really intimate experience, even if it is not sexual. Part of the reason that it is so intimate is that you are working outside of the confines of your comfort to bring your partner pleasure. When you give your partner a massage, you are focusing on their pleasure, rather than your pleasure, which in turn can bring you joy knowing that you are satisfying the needs of your partner.

A lot of people shy away from giving their partner massages because they feel they are not skilled enough to give a massage. The truth is, you do not have to be an expert to make your partner feel good. A lot of the times it is the caring and loving touches you give that make a massage feel good. Communicate and find a good pressure to start out with, and encourage your partner to tell you what does and does not feel good, so that you can give them a good massage that leaves them feeling relaxed.

Oils

First of all, find an oil that is lightly scented, and prepare it for the massage. You should only oil the section that you are working on at present for the oil not to absorb into the skin before you make it to that portion of the body.

When applying a massage oil, you should always warm it up between your hands before applying it to the skin so that it is warm rather than cold. Cold oil will be a shock to the skin and is not really pleasant in a massage. However, when warmed up, massage oils create a pleasant sensation on the skin and body that will leave your lover trembling with pleasure.

How to Massage

Always start with your partner laying on their stomach. Start at their feet, and using a downward motion, massage their feet. Be sure to use a gentle touch, and take your time. Devote your attention to one foot at a time, massaging from the toes down to the heel. Spend a little extra time focusing on the arch of the foot, as that is where a lot of the tension in the feet build up at.

Once you have massaged each foot, you can then move up to the calves. Again, using soft downwards strokes, massage each calf individually. Start at the sides, and work your way to the top. When you get to the highest point on the calf, switch to circular motions to un-knot any tense muscles that may reside there. Again, take your time, and don't rush to get to the next part of the body, as you want your partner to be fully satisfied.

Now you can move onto the back of the thighs. The thighs are one of the more sensitive areas of the body, so avoid tickling your partner. You may need to use a little more pressure here to do so. Just like with the calves, start from the sides, and work your way up using downward motions. Work on each leg separately, and really focus on the outer part of the thigh, where a lot of the tension resides due to those muscles doing a lot of the work throughout the day.

If you think that you were going to skip the buttocks, you are entirely wrong. The buttocks are a very sensual area of the body and deserve attention devoted to them as well. You want to use circular motions here, and a little more pressure. Squeezing and rubbing are also acceptable here. You want to pay attention to both cheeks separately, just like with the legs and feet. Take your time and really worship the bottom.

Now you can move on to the parts of the body most people equate with massages. The back, shoulders, and neck. However, you should pay attention to each part individually, and give each your undivided attention. Start with the small of the back, right where it meets the buttocks, and the side/hip area. Starting at the sides, work your way into the middle. Be careful if your partner is ticklish here. You may have to increase the pressure a little to make it less tickling. Slowly slide up the back and massage between the small of the back and the shoulder blades. Again, start with the sides and work your way to the top. You can use a variety of motions on this portion of the body, such as a hacking karate chop, an almost poking motion with the balls of your fingers, or a cupping motion where you push on the back with cupped hands. Makes sure not to do any of these too hard, just enough to relax the muscles in the back.

Now you can move on to the shoulder blade area. This area often holds a lot of tension and can really create a lot of pleasure once that tension is released. Pick a motion that feels good for your partner, and really focus on in between the shoulder blades before moving onto the shoulders and neck.

Moving to the front of your partner, you want to use feather like touches. Massage the arms first, and then the front of the shoulders. Massage each arm separately and the front of the shoulders together. Slowly work your way down to the sides of the breasts, and the ribcage. These are really erogenous areas, so be sure to spend extra time on them, massaging the oils in well. Move up the rib cage and up between the breasts. Massage the sides of the breasts, working up to the nipples, and back down to the abdomen. You want to make sure that you are using light strokes, but not too light. The idea is to relax your partner's muscles, not tease them.

Work your way down the stomach to the navel area. Focus on that spot especially. It is very sensitive, and can really get your partner going. Slowly work your way down the navel to the front of the thighs, and using the same techniques as the back of the legs work down to the feet, and back up to the genital area. From here you can choose just to massage or to stimulate the genital area as you please.

Foreplay is an important part of lovemaking, and it is essential that you employ it at least occasionally to really spice up your love life.

Let's state the obvious: foreplay is amazing. It's the preview of what's about to happen, the prologue to an amazing romantic evening, the teaser if you will. This chapter will cover a few techniques lovers can implement to entice and tease one another, to set the mood, and drive each other into a sexual frenzy.

It's important to highlight one very simple, but somehow overlooked fact, in most relationships: Flirting doesn't stop once you're in a relationship! Flirting and seduction are as important to a love life as much as genitals, tongues, breasts, and other body parts! It's not just for folks that are dating one another, not just for young people, not just for horny couples that are just experiencing their partner's body for the first time. This is a theme that will be repeated throughout this text, the spark lights the fire. And there's nothing better to get that spark raging than teasing, touching, and a whole lot of foreplay. Remember, the Kama Sutra is more about the art of seducing your love than just a bunch of sex positions (although those positions are important!). Other highlights in this chapter will include talking about sending sexy pictures or texts or emails, phone calls, little notes, setting the tone for an evening or day of lovemaking, tips for oral sex, kissing, and things of that nature.

So, now that we have you all worked up, let's get down to it!

Teasing

The art of the tease cannot be understated. Strippers understand it. Burlesque dancers understand it. Lingerie clothing manufacturers understand it. Heck, even the producers of mainstream, big-budget films understand it when they're putting together a trailer for a film they want you to spend money to see this summer! So, how can we draw upon these mediums and get a complete understanding of what teasing's all about?

Well, first off, let's examine one fundamental aspect of teasing. Much like what we said about foreplay, the tease should be a preview. It's the one thing that can get the blood flowing to all of those *ahem* important parts of the body. A quick tease can be a great way to let your lover know that what's going to take place later will blow their minds!

Teasing, obviously, can take many different forms. Leaving a little note, or series of notes, around the house before leaving for work, letting your significant other know what you plan on doing to them, and with them, later on, is a surefire way to get someone's heart racing. Guys, wouldn't you like to wake up one day to get ready for work to see that your wife, who's already left for the day, has left you a note saying, "I can't wait to put my lips on you," or, ladies, what if a man left a little note in your purse that said, "Be naked when I get home." This may be a case of overstating it bluntly or obviously, but most of us would kill for little notes like that.

Texts or emails are great too. Quick little texts that can either be coy, ("I can't wait to show you what I bought at Adam & Eve") middle of the road, ("I can't stop touching myself thinking about you") or downright triple-X ("I'm going to lick your tight, wet pussy later"). If you know what your partner likes in terms of dirty talk, erotic words, and the like, then send them what they want to hear. If you're at the beginning of the relationship and still feeling them out (no pun intended), then try all of them. But, remember, it's called a tease for a reason. Don't go overboard here. Don't sit down with your cell phone in your hand and start working on the first chapter of an erotic novel that would make Larry Flynt or Jenna Jameson blush. Keep it simple, keep it quick. Even just a few words will suffice. And if you're sending pics (nude, topless, bottomless, dick pics, whatever) one or two will also suffice. "Brevity is the soul of wit," as William Shakespeare once noted, but it's also the essence of a good tease.

Also, please keep in mind that when sending a text or an email or whatever you choose to send, your partner has to be alone, or have some type of privacy when viewing it or responding to it. When two people are riled up and ready for an evening of sex, sometimes their senses and better judgments can get clouded. Don't send an email to your partner's work email. Don't send the text when you know they're in a meeting or if you know they're around a whole host of co-workers. Yes, orgasms are amazing, and yes, seeing your partner sexually satisfied and happy, and content is a great feeling, but you don't want to risk someone's job or livelihood over it. Keep your cool, and tease when you can!

Watching Porn

Some couples love watching porn together. It's a great way to get each other in the mood. Watching another couple or couples have amazing sex while pleasuring their amazing bodies, with amazing techniques, is...well, amazing! If you and your partner love sharing this experience together, why wait? Get to it, then! However, if your partner is unsure about watching with another person, (because let's face it, some of us would rather watch it alone, or have watched it alone for so long that we can't entertain the notion of watching with another person) suggest it to them, but like anything else discussed here, don't pressure them into accepting it.

If you and your partner do decide to watch porn to get yourselves really worked up, the internet (to absolutely no one's surprise) has literally millions of sites to choose from, with hundreds of different categories: girl-girl, BBW, gay, orgy, busty, well hung, interracial, etc. Of course, if you want to go the more traditional route, an adult video store will also have many genres and titles to choose from. And since many people nowadays watch their porn on the internet, many adult video and bookstores have numerous DVDs and Blu-Rays for discounted prices. It's not uncommon to find a compilation film, or even a classic adult film (like Behind the Green Door, or Debbie Does Dallas) for a very affordable price.

Novelties

Novelties are a great way to introduce a little fun in the bedroom! Whether you pick up a pair of adult dice ('Kiss'/ 'Neck'/ 'Lick' / 'Below Waist') or a pair of handcuffs, these can enhance the naughtiness and help put a smile on your face... in a variety of ways, if you catch our drift.

Toys

Aside from a penis, a tongue, or fingers, a vibrator can be a woman's best friend. If you're a woman that doesn't have a vibrator (you poor, deprived thing!), you might want to consider getting one. Not only is it a great masturbation tool and a fine stress reliever, but it's also a wonderful way to share a sexual experience with your partner. Vibrators come in a variety of different shapes, sizes, styles, etc. You can get the old school, white plastic model, or you can go for the ultra-realistic looking dildo in the shape and size of your favorite male porn star.

If you're a little too shy to step into a store to pick one up, you can always order one online from numerous different websites. But, trust us, if you need some assistance in choosing one, or want some advice on which to go with, it's probably best to just take the plunge and step into a store. The people who work in the store are there to help you. Get rid of any sort of notion that you might have of someone criticizing you or making fun of you. They won't do that in the slightest. At the end of the day, their store is no different from any other retail outlet or business. They sell things people want or need, and they stay in business for a reason: supply and demand.

And shopping for toys such as vibrators, nipple clamps, nipple vibrators, or male sex toys (like masturbation sleeves, or pocket pussies) can do what we've mentioned and will keep mentioning throughout this book repeatedly, it brings a couple closer together. When two people take an active role and figure out what kind of toy or toys they'd like to utilize to spice up the sex, it can be a great and rewarding experience.

Massages are important

If there was ever a gateway to amazing sex, it has to be a massage. Lying down, naked or half-naked, your partner's warm hands rubbing your body, relaxing you, touching you... It's enough to make one want to hop in bed and get off just thinking about it. If you or your partner have never massaged each other, now is the time to try it out yourselves. As stated, it's a brilliant way to get each other worked up and to get in the mood, and it can lead to a night of sensual sex.

If your partner likes it a little rough, then make sure to work the muscles and the skin a bit harder. If your partner prefers a soft touch, then lightly move your hands over their body, head to toe and in all points in between. And, don't forget, a happy ending is preferred!

Baths and Showers

Water can be a stimulating thing. Having a warm liquid all over your body can get the blood flowing and the heart racing (two things that a very intricate to sexual arousal). Two people relaxing naked and wet in a tub together is glorious. It's a perfect way to begin the act of foreplay. Maybe take it one step further and light a few candles. Play some soft music. And, most importantly, wash each other! Take a washcloth or a soft sponge and maneuver it all over your lover's body. The sensual touching, the warm water, the steam, all of it can lull a person into a perfect state of relaxation. While your hands are under the water, slowly move them to your partner's legs, work inward, and begin touching them. Stroke his penis slowly, play with her clitoris lightly. Kiss their neck, nibble on their ears, lick their nipples, and bring them right to the edge.

Foreplay

Most women will agree on one thing: when it comes to foreplay, it sometimes doesn't last nearly long enough as it should. It might sound cliché, but women are like a stove and men are like a microwave. A guy, especially a younger man, is 'ready to go' at a moment's notice, whereas a woman would like things to progress a little slower. With this in mind, it's a good idea to take your time, guys. Don't rush it. Keep your cool. Know that a wonderful release is waiting at the end of a great night of sex. But it's not a race! Slow down there. Just enjoy the scenery. Explore every inch of her incredible body.

Here are some tips for making your foreplay experience a little more pleasurable:

• Oral

Do it. And then do it some more. Straight ladies and gay men, learn to give a great blowjob. Straight men and gay ladies, learn to eat pussy. Just take your time. Pay attention to your lover's body. If they're moaning, if their body is writhing, if they're grabbing your hair and trying to pull your head even closer to their body, then you are certainly doing something right. Guys, most women can climax multiple times throughout a lovemaking session, so learn, learn, learn the art of cunnilingus. Lick and suck on her clit, insert a finger or two inside of her (palm up, making a 'come here' motion with your fingers, teasing her G-Spot), and make her cum hard!

• Nipple Play

Again, do it! Most women absolutely love to have their nipples played with, tugged, licked, sucked, nibbled, and sometimes bitten, or all of the above. And here's a little secret, guys do as well. Most gay men already know the pleasures of nipple play, but many straight guys don't. Ladies, pay as much attention to your man's nipples as he does yours. Also, there's a common misconception out there that busty ladies tend to not have as sensitive nipples as ladies with a smaller bust, but that's not always the case. Just because a woman has bigger boobs doesn't mean she's dead in that area. So, lick and suck to your heart's content!

- Anal and Anal Play

Obviously, this is an area where your partner has to feel comfortable playing with. For some women, it just doesn't feel right, and some guys don't like that have that area touched, teased, or played with. But if your partner does, then learn to up your anal game. Learn to give great rim jobs, and learn how to slowly insert your fingers or penis with generous amounts of lube. Speaking of which...

- Body butter and flavored lubes

Lube can be your friend, so don't skimp on it. Whether you get water-based lube, the flavored kind for all of the licking and sucking you plan to do, or whether you get the warming kind to add a little heat to the situation, it's always a good idea to keep some around. Saliva is the best form of lube that there is, but for those of you who want to try anal or something along the lines of titty-fucking, lubricant is your best bet. You can pick up lots of different lubes at your local sex shop or adult bookstore, and you can even get a few varieties at places such as Walmart, Rite Aid, or Walgreens.

- Food

This might be a turn off for some, but for others adding a little chocolate or whipped cream or ice cubes to the bedroom is amazing. Licking warm chocolate off of your girl's clit can be a treat for both of you! And for some ladies, the feeling of an ice cube being rubbed slowly against her nipples can send them over the edge! Obviously, discuss it with your partner first before bringing in a tray of food. You don't want to turn them off.

- Spanking

Some people like it and some don't. If you're a person that does, and your partner doesn't, gently ask if they'll do that for you. If you're the one that likes to spank, and your partner doesn't, maybe give no more than a tap or two on the butt. Again, talk with your partner, and refer back to chapter one. You don't want to go full tilt gonzo and delve into a dom/sub S and M relationship when your partner doesn't want anything to do with it.

- Talking Dirty

Talking dirty can enhance the passion, and make the lovemaking even more intense. If your partner doesn't like an overt amount of swearing or gets offended at some choice words, maybe you should avoid this, but don't let that stop you from talking. If you don't want to delve into the dirty talk, then just speak calmly and happily. Compliment her body. Moan in appreciation. Tell him he's amazing. Tell her that she's beautiful. When your lover hears what they're doing right, they'll do more of it. When they hear that you think they're gorgeous, it will spike their confidence. And when the two of you are locked in that respective situation and airing your appreciation and love for one another, your relationship deepens.

• 	Kissing and Touching

This one should be obvious enough. Kissing on the lips, or touching someone on those special places on a person's body, is the fast track to arousal. In other words, you are stimulating the erogenous zones. Most sex therapists and scientists agree that there are seven main erogenous zones for female and male bodies.

For women, these include the clitoris, vagina, cervix, mouth, neck, ears, and nipples. For men, it's the penis, scrotum, mouth, neck, ears, nipples, and perineum (the space between a man's scrotum and anus, which can also be called, in basic terminology, the 'taint'). However, did you know that the erogenous zones don't stop there? Try kissing or lightly touching the shoulders, the upper part of the back, the inside part of the arm on the opposite side of the elbow, the back of the knee, and, if you're willing and if your partner is into it, the feet, especially the toes. Everyone is built differently.

A woman's nipples may not be as sensitive as, say, her neck. Or a guy's scrotum may be way, way, way too sensitive to even touch or play with, and may make him feel uncomfortable if you do so. But, you see, this can actually be part of the fun! If you take your time and move your mouth and hands on to all parts of your lovers' body, you become familiar with what turns them on and drives them crazy, and you learn what areas to avoid.

• Nudism

This can be a fun and pleasant activity! Pick a day, or an afternoon, or any part, throughout the day, and just be naked! Do whatever it is that you would normally do (chores, cleaning, cooking, sitting down together and watching television, reading, etc.,) but do it completely naked. And if you have a large yard with neighbors that live quite a ways away, spend some time outside in the nude.

If you have a pool, go skinny dipping! Do anything you'd like without any clothes on whatsoever. This can help in many different ways. Granted, the act of going out naked is not explicitly sexual, but it can lead to a round of teasing later on.

And, let's face it, the sight of your lover doing a task or just sitting there in the nude can be a nice scene to get your blood flowing. And, finally, the more naked that you and your partner are on a more regular basis, the more and more comfortable you'll be in your own skins! As we've stated before and will state again before the book is over, confidence is a turn on. Confident people believe in themselves. And when you believe in yourself, you make yourself even more attractive to your partner, thus enhancing the foreplay and sex that's sure to come (much like you and your partner, no pun intended) later on.

Touching! Teasing! Talking! Licks, nibbles, scents, and playing! Remember, everyone, slow down, take your time, and enjoy the hell out of your foreplay.

More than Just Sex

Kissing and embracing are almost as important as foreplay. In fact, they could be considered types of foreplay, but as they can also be used in intimacy that does not involve sex, they are in their own section. These are really important parts of being intimate with your partner, even on a regular basis, so they should not be overlooked. If you feel like the love is dying in your relationship, try some of these tips for reasons other than sex, and you will find that the passion is reignited. The love isn't gone, your romance is just not as robust as it used to be.

Kissing and mouth play

Kissing is an inherent part of our culture. In nearly every movie or show you see, there is a kiss of some sort. Even action movies often have a kiss and a love story plot line. In relationships, the excitement builds as you go in for that first kiss. Sometimes it is awkward, and sometimes it is passionate and perfect, but nonetheless, you love it anyway. Kissing is just that ingrained in our culture. While we are not the only species to kiss, we are the only species to do so with the passion and intensity that we do. So why hide the evolutionary perks, and be stingy with kisses?

There are several different types of kisses out there. These kisses range from gentle, loving kisses to steamy, passionate kisses. You want to use these kisses in your everyday life with your partner. Maybe not all of them in the same day, but mix it up a little bit. There is more to the kissing scene than just the peck or the simple French kiss. Even if you try one of these and it seems a little sloppy, you can always try again. Just like with sexual positions, some take practice to get down.

Starting with the soft kisses that are great for everyday use here are a few.

 Eyelash Kiss: This is great for people with long eyelashes. It may seem a little awkward at first if you have not attempted it before, but after a while, it will leave you wanting more. The partner with the long eyelashes brushes their eyelashes against their partner's lips. You want to make sure that you do it lightly and briefly, to really create an intimate encounter.

Forehead Kiss: This is a kiss that shows love and tenderness. This kiss is used to show that you will be there for a person, and that you care for them. Often also used to comfort a lover who is upset or scared. These kisses, while simple are very intimate and loving.

Awakening Kiss: The awakening kiss is used by one lover to awaken their sleeping partner. It can be applied gently to the temple, or to the lips. This is a really light, gently kiss that increases slightly in pressure at the end. This tender kiss is designed to wake your partner up lovingly so that they start the day on a good note. This should be used every morning, not just on mornings you want a little amorous fun.

Public Kiss: For those who are a little afraid to show public affection, fret not. This kiss does not mean you have a tongue war in the middle of the street, it refers to a simple kiss on the hand or the neck, just to let the world know that your partner is taken, and to make your partner feel special in a crowd of so many people.

Throbbing Kiss: This is a series of light, small kisses. These kisses are playful and fun, but also convey love and emotion. They are a great way to initiate a little more fun, and more intense kisses, as well as just some goodnight kisses when you don't want to say goodnight, but you have to.

Goodbye Kiss: This is a special kind of kiss that you give your lover when you leave. This kiss is intimate, but can also leave them thinking about you until you return. This kiss is slow and passionate, and is followed by a gesture that will embed itself in your partner's mind all day. Start by kissing your partner slowly and deeply, and then as the kiss finishes, place your index and middle fingers together on your partner's lips as you depart. This is a lingering kiss that will make both of you think about each other.

Now time for the steamy kisses that are out there. There are several kisses that you can use to ignite a passion in your lover that will drive them wild and can lead to more adult pleasures.

Distracting Kiss: This is a kiss that you use to distract your lover from what they are doing. This will peak their interest, and they will love the spontaneity. (As long as they are not doing something super important.) To do this kiss, simply find a spot on the body that is sensitive, such as the earlobe or neck, and kiss on that spot until they turn their head. Once they turn their face to you, take their lips and kiss them passionately. This is guaranteed to drive them wild.

Kiss with a Finger: This is an alluring kiss that is an open invitation for oral sex. This steamy kiss can be seen as a little awkward at first, but once you get into it, it can be really enticing. This kiss involves putting your finger in your partner's mouth and letting them suck on it, and then taking it out. Once you take your finger out, rub it across your lips while looking into their eyes. You could possibly even wink if you can do so in a sultry manner. It is definitely a kiss to get you thinking about sex.

Corner Kiss: It's a simple kiss that can seem really innocent, but the passion below is something else. You will find that using this kiss can lead to a lot more passionate and deep kisses, so use this kiss with caution. This is a kiss that occurs at the corners of the mouth, and drive both you and your partner wild, because the subtle hint of sexy leaves you wanting so much more. When you are doing this kiss, be sure to make it short and light, yet also very intense. It will do wonders for starting a flame going.

Clip Kiss: This is a simple, yet passionate kiss that you may have already tried in your life. However, if you haven't, you definitely have to try it, because it will definitely spice up the way you kiss your partner. This is one of the deeper kisses, and it is fun, flirty, and sensual. With this kiss, you gently touch your partner's lips or tongue with the tip of your tongue. This will send you both into a pleasurable little tongue battle that can lead to a lot more than just simple kissing.

Top Kiss: This is fun and sensual kiss that is used by a lot of people, but is deemed a little intense. This involves taking the top lip of your partner gently in your teeth and sucking on it while they do the same with your bottom lip. This is great coupled with some tongue to start the progression on into foreplay. Be careful not to bite too hard with this kiss. While a little pain is often pleasurable, sharp pain is almost guaranteed to ruin the mood, and you do not want the mood to be ruined.

Bent Kiss: This one can be romantic as well as steamy. This is a simple kiss that is not too sloppy or messy and can actually be emotionally charged. It is a good use for when one partner is taller than the other, or when they are at different angles. This kiss involves one partner tilting their lover's head back, and holding the chin in their hand. Then, the first partner kisses their love's upturned lips gently and sweetly. This is a great kiss for slow and passionate sex, as it is emotionally charged, and sets the tone nicely.

Those are some great kisses to use on your partner to try to reignite the passion in your relationship. These kisses are perfect at any time, or also to get things started in a little more amorous manner. There is more to passion than kissing though. In foreplay, the mouth can be a very useful tool.

Many people underestimate the power of a well-placed kiss, nibble, or lick. The truth is, these are an essential part of intimate lovemaking. You want to make sure that you employ these techniques all along your partner's body, because there are so many erogenous zones, and most of them do not get a lot of attention because most people don't know about them.

The Back

The back is actually a very erogenous zone. There are so many nerve endings in the back, and if used well, they can entice and excite a lover to the highest extremes. You want to take your time, and really focus on the back. Of course, there are massages, but you want to use your mouth on the back too.

Try lightly kissing your partner between the shoulder blades, and increasing the pressure of your kisses down their spine to the small of their back. You can follow the kisses by trailing your fingers down their spine. Move your lips to each side and intensify your kisses by pulling the skin between your teeth and sucking. Do not really bite here, as the skin can be very sensitive. Sucking can create an intense pleasure, though. Follow back up to the shoulder blade, again trailing your fingers after. Then move over to the other side and go back down sucking with your mouth and lightly brushing with your fingers. Follow back up the line of kisses down the spine.

You can do this once, or repeat several times if you would like. However, if you choose to repeat, it is a good idea to take a break between each time to do something else to create a tantalizing feeling and to ensure that you are not causing pain by sucking the same spots over and over again.

Shoulders

The shoulders are another sensitive area on the body, particularly right where they meet with the neck. This is a great spot to place love bites and kisses along. A lot of people think that biting is a little too extreme, and not for them. However, you will find that biting gently in the right areas can bring your partner some intense pleasure. Some people can almost get off just by being nipped in the right area.

The shoulders are one of the best areas for love bites, as they are strong, and the skin there is tough. They are also sensitive enough that the pressure from a gentle bite creates a massive amount of pleasure. When you apply a love bite, make sure that you are not biting too hard, but also hard enough to create heightened pleasure. Apply a medium pressure to your bite. If your lover tries to pull their neck in to stop you, decrease the pressure and try again. The best place for love bites is right at the back of the neck where it meets the shoulders or right at the sides. If your partner is laying on their back, the collar bone is also a pleasurable place for a love bite. Always follow the bite with a gentle kiss, as if soothing the area.

Chapter 3: Sex

As stated in the introduction to this book, most people think that the Kama Sutra is filled with nothing but pictures and illustrations of sex, and as we've established, it doesn't encompass the entirety of the book. However, it is a very important aspect. In this chapter, we will take a look at a few different positions that couples can try, where to try them when to try them, as well as other parts and pieces that can enhance your sex life and bring yourself to a deep understanding of pleasure and how to achieve it.

We will continue on by explaining certain sex positions, but please understand we are really only scraping the surface when it comes to the discussion of these positions. The Kama Sutra has 64 positions, and we will, for the sake of brevity and the space allotted here in this book, take a look at a handful of them. And the following positions that we will examine are the 'beginner' positions. For a more in-depth look at the other positions, please find a copy of the Kama Sutra itself and dive right in!

Various Kama Sutra Sex Positions

The Congress of the Crow

This one is basically the same as the better known '69' position, except the two lovers, lie on their sides, instead of one lying on their back while the other straddles their lover. This is a great one to start off with because you're pretty much moving from teasing, to foreplay, to this position. It's a perfect start to intense lovemaking.

As stated, lie on your side with your head facing toward your partner's genitals, and begin to pleasure them orally. If need be, spread the legs for better access. And you can stay in this position for quite a while, or you can move into the traditional 69. For those that prefer oral over actual sex, or for the ladies who find it hard to cum through penetration, this is a wonderful position.

The Clasping Position

This one is quite similar to the 'missionary' position, however, instead of staying on his knees, the man enters the woman and soon after penetration, stretches his legs outward, as the does the woman beneath him.

This also works for the woman on top. After her man enters her, she adjusts her body and stretches her legs out in the very same manner. This is a great way for a woman to take control of the situation! She can adjust the speed and depth of the penetration to suit her needs.

Tigress

Almost like the 'reverse cowgirl,' there are a few very minor differences between that position and the tigress position. The woman mounts the man, facing in the opposite direction (much like Reverse Cowgirl) but instead of staying on her knees, she stays on her feet. This is a good one for the more flexible ladies.

(If you do have a hard time bending down, or staying in that position for a long time, this is one that you might want to skip.)

Another aspect of the tigress is that the woman, while still facing away from her man, reaches back with one hand and can either rest it on his chest or stimulate his nipples. All in all, if you have the agility and limber legs, the one technique that's sure to hit all of the right spots (inside and out) with the ladies!

Splitting the Bamboo

Again, much in the same way that the 'clasping' position draws heavily from the 'missionary' position, 'splitting the bamboo' allows the woman to lie down and let the man do the work. The difference here is the fact that the woman raises one leg and rests it on the man's shoulder, chest, or somewhere near his head. This allows for deeper penetration, and it lets the guy control the speed and thrust of the situation.

Alternate from leg to leg. Raise your right one, and then switch to the left, and then back again. Or raise both at the same time. You'd be surprised at how these tiny little adjustments can add another level of pleasure!

Tripadam (Or Tripod)

This position requires the two of you to stand and face each other. The woman raises one leg up, the man holds that one leg with his hand, enters the woman, and they have sex until they reach their climax, standing the whole time. The two can either stand without any sort of support, or they can lean against a wall.

Really, this one is recommended for people of respective height. If your man is tall and you're petite, this one might be a pass, unless you want to find something to stand on and engage in some impressive balancing.

The Curled Angel

Lie on your sides in a cuddling, spooning position... and then fuck! Really, that's all there is to this one. But, let's be open and honest about one thing: for certain body types, this one might have to be avoided. Bigger people might have a hard time interlocking in this position, and guys who aren't blessed with a long one probably can't reach the vagina. But, if you can do it, then do it you must!

71

Rocking Horse

Again, the woman is on top of this one. It's much like the traditional cowgirl position in the sense that the woman is on her knees, atop her man, facing him, but the guy leans up and draws his body closer to the lady at an almost 45-degree angle. This is a good one for deep penetration and to allow the woman to control every single aspect of the lovemaking.

The Padlock

This is a great one. The woman sits on the edge of a surface, a bed, a couch, whatever, angling her body so that the man, who stands, can enter her easily. The man is in control for this one, and the fact that he's able to stay on his feet gives him the chance to enhance his speed and thrusting ability.

Doggy

This one goes by various names (depending on the translation), but we're going to go ahead and let the common terminology do the talking. Chances are, you already know this one. If you haven't done it yourself, you've probably seen it in porn.

The woman is on her knees, facing away from the man, and the man enters her from behind. The great aspect of the 'doggy' style is the fact that both the man and the woman can control the speed by working in tandem together! Also, by using his hands, the man can give little taps and slaps on the woman's butt if she's into spanking. Or, he can maneuver one hand in front of him, reach down between the woman's legs, and stimulate her clit while still thrusting away. Or, both hands can slide their way up to her breasts, cup them, squeeze them, and play with them.

Again, please keep in mind these examples are only a minor taste of what you can find in the Kama Sutra. After you've tried these positions, and some of the other ideas and tips mentioned in this book, please consider picking up a copy. Trust us, you won't be sorry that you did!

Kinks and Fetishes

When we hear the words 'kink' or 'fetish' it usually invokes images of leather-clad people spanking and beating one another with whips, chains, and cat-o-nine tails. Although those types of outfits and actions and implements can indeed fall into the category of a kink or a fetish, they aren't exclusive. One big aspect of sex and sexuality is to understand the fundamental difference between what is known as a kink and what is called a fetish. Some people the world over tend to think that both of them fall into the same category and that's not the case.

A kink is defined as being something that you really like and want to have somewhere in the spectrum while you're having sex, or masturbating, but if that particular thing, whatever it may be, isn't there, you can still have fun and achieve orgasm. For instance, let's say a kink of yours is to gaze at a nice, big, round ass, or a very large bust of a woman. But if you happen to be with a woman with a flat or not as plump backside or smaller boobs, you'll still have fun and get off with no problems whatsoever. You enjoy the person, appreciate their body, and love cumming with them.

A fetish, however, is a little deeper. This is the thing that you need, that you crave, that you absolutely must have while having sex or masturbating to achieve any sort of fun at all. If you're into the aforementioned round butt or big boobs to the point that you need to have them to cum, then you have a fetish for those body areas.

Understanding these two things, and understanding it with your significant other, will allow you to explore the parameters of what you're into, in terms of sexual desire, just a little bit further.

Location, Location, Location

We've spoken before about how the Kama Sutra is filled with descriptions of turning a certain section of your home into a love chamber or a chamber of love. But one of the hottest things you can do to add a jolt of energy to your sex life is to have sex in other parts of your home. Don't just keep it in the bedroom. Again, explore and experiment!

Try having sex in the living room or even in the kitchen. If you haven't yet tried making love in the bathtub, how about a nice round of oral sex in the hallway? How about outside?

If you live with other people, have a few kids around the house, or have neighbors that live well within earshot, maybe consider getting a hotel for a night or two, or renting a cottage somewhere.

Anything that you can do to add some spark to your love life is sure to help make the experience better!

Time and Time Again

We've discussed techniques, methods, and location. Now we need to talk about the times throughout the day when to have sex. Well...any time is great for some of us. But if you're more of a wait-until-the-end-of-the-day kind of person, maybe flip the script and surprise your lover with some hot morning sex before starting the day. Or, if you two happened to take a lunch break from your respective jobs at the same time, and if time permits, how about a little side dish of oral sex and missionary with your lunch? Some people think it's hot to get stirred awake in the middle of the night by the hands and lips of your lover. There you are, sleeping, dreaming, and then after a few seconds of being pulled from your slumber, you feel kisses on your neck and a hand manipulating that special spot between your legs. There's a meme that you can find on the internet that says something to the effect of "You have my permission to wake me up if you're horny!" Let this apply itself to you as well!

When it comes to foreplay, sex, arousal, and all that's involved with making your love life even better than what it is, all you have to do is to take the time to find the time to do it. And then find some more time after that.

Cumming

Let's talk about it. Some straight women and gay men don't like getting it on them, some don't mind at all. Some people swallow, others spit, some can go either way. Some want nothing to do with facials. Some love it. Whatever your preference is, talk it over with your man. If he's totally into facials and it really gets him excited, consider it. But if it's a no-go, then gently explain it to him. Once more, yet again, for the umpteenth time, communication is key.

When it comes to, well, cum, it's the finish line, the end zone, the home plate. Get there with each other, and have fun doing so!

If It Doesn't Happen...

But there's a chance that it doesn't go off the way you planned, and it could be because of the fact that your partner went off way too early.

Whatever it is, don't fret. If you tried some of these tips and are still falling short of that finish line, end zone, home plate, again, talk it over. Tell your lover what you're missing. Be sure to compliment them on what they're good at, but if you're still missing that essential spark, you have to speak up. Don't let your personal pleasure go without, and don't keep your desires to yourself. Share, speak, talk, communicate with your significant other!

Other Ways and Means

Before we move on, we must also address one additional item concerning sex, not every round of lovemaking needs to be a well-planned, thought out, discussed, diagrammed, and timed thing! Spontaneous sex is also hot! Imagine coming home from work one day and you see your partner on the couch completely naked.

And within a few seconds, you are too. A few minutes and one orgasm later, you feel relaxed and ready to eat supper, and you continue on with your evening like normal.

Quickies are fun. And, trust us, they're not just the preferred method for men. Women like them as well! If it's a choice between going a full twenty-four hours without any hint of sex or getting off, or finding a quick five minutes to cum, most of us are without a doubt going to choose the later.

And then there are three-ways... it should be noted, that this is something that, out of all of the things mentioned in this book, needs to be discussed, discussed, discussed, and discussed some more. Although most men and some women do have a three-way fantasy circling in their heads from time to time (or, for some, almost all of the time), the finer details need to be talked about, pored over, dissected, and examined. Would your partner really be okay with a third party coming into the fray? Would you? Would you end up getting jealous? Would this result in a serious problem down the road?

Let's state one thing, watching a three-way on film is ridiculously hot. It's over the top in its eroticism. If you're a woman who loves the sight of a well-chiseled, well-hung man, then what's better than having two of them? And if you're a guy that loves young, tanned, curvy women, seeing two of them pleasure a guy in almost any form imaginable is a sight to behold for sure. But just because it works on screen, or in the pictorials of a magazine, doesn't mean it's for everyone. Most of us don't want to share our love with someone else. Some of us would freak out like crazy if we saw someone kissing them, touching them, or taking their clothes off. But some of us love this idea! If you do, and you want to explore it further, again, talk it out. Walk yourselves through it. Lay down some ground rules. For instance, some couples put a restriction on who joins them in the bedroom, e.g., it can't be a friend of ours, it can't be someone we work with, etc. Some have a restriction on what can be done with, and to, that third person, e.g., no actual penetration, oral only, or everything is fair game for all involved, etc.

Whatever the ins and outs are, take note of them. Make sure to set the standards and rules and stick to them!

And when speaking of sex we should also talk about the most familiar form of sex that just about every living mammal on planet Earth experiences more of than anything, and that, of course, is masturbation. Masturbating, aside from sex with someone you love and care deeply for, is the single greatest form of pleasure there is. And, if you haven't already, try mutual masturbation with your partner. Kiss, tease, get naked, and then watch each other. Watch how your partner's hands work their body. Watch them as they cum. And expose yourself to being watched as well. Or, if you like, sit side by side and watch an adult movie, or clips on the internet. The fact is, masturbating (or 'jerking' off, or 'frigging,' or 'beating' off, or whatever the preferred slang term it is that you want to use) is a private thing. It's personal. And, for most of us, it's been our go-to stress reliever and sexual conduit since we were teenagers, or pre-teens even. We slip beneath the covers or go to the restroom, cell phone in hand with an internet site with our favorite porn queued up, or magazine, or an overactive imagination, and we go to town! So, taking the time to share that part of our lives and ourselves with another person is just another way of letting someone see the deeper part of ourselves. It's another form of sharing our bodies, our souls, our lusts, our likes, our needs with someone we love.

And everything that we've spoken about thus far is exactly that. It's not just about inserting one area of the body into someone else's body, it's about giving yourself, every part of yourself freely, and allowing yourself, every part of yourself, to be taken by another. Physical sex is amazing, make no mistake. But having

81

that physical connection, that spiritual, emotional, and mental connection with another and then letting those connections grow to newer and better heights are things that cannot simply be put into words.

Chapter 4: Making Yourself Attractive

Let's face it. As much as we would like to think that we're enlightened, cultured, and sometimes above surface-level ideas, at our root, at the core, we're all sexual beings who are looking to get off. We crave flesh. We need to cum. And we love the visual appeal of a person that we find attractive. And there's nothing better, or more erotic, than seeing a person that we're in love with all dressed up, cleaned up, and made up. It appeals to all of our senses and plays with our libido. It's the very thing that sets us on a course toward orgasm.

There are a number of ways that we can make ourselves more attractive to our significant others, and most of these ways deal with tantalizing our basic human senses: touch, taste, sight, smell, and hearing. Those senses are at the center of who we are, and to get your partner, and yourself, in the mood, it's best to not just pay attention to one or a few of those senses. Tease all of them!

First, let's talk about possibly the strongest sense that most of us have...

Scent

Scent is one of the strongest senses we have, and as many women can attest, there's nothing that can tease them faster than a man who wears a nice smelling cologne, or a woman who knows how to dab on a perfect scent.

Psychologists have, for over a century, documented the importance of the sense of smell. Smell is usually the first sign of danger, whether it's an odd smell in a home or the scent of a fire in the distance. But it can also have a calming, easing, effect on us. When our olfactory senses are relaxed, so are we. When those senses are teased, well, so are we. Perfume and cologne makers understand this better than most people. After all, they've built a multi-million dollar industry that has been a constantly growing for century after century. Frankly, not many industries on the planet can lay claim to that.

Perfume making is one of the oldest types of industry in the world. Its roots are older than most established countries, governments, and religions, and can be found in scripts and texts from ancient China, India, and Mesopotamia. In fact, the world's oldest chemist who delved into the art of making finer scents for wearable purposes was a woman by the name of Tapputi, an overseer of the royal palace of Mesopotamia and a governmental figure of her time. Many of her techniques have been passed down through generations of perfume and cologne makers, and the very basis of what she implemented is still used to this day.

By the medieval period, France and Italy became the leaders in perfume making, and by the Victorian Era, England had become a respected maker as well. Today, many fine cologne and perfume companies, such as Mäurer & Wirtz and Floris of London, have been around for many years and have been long regarded as industry leaders.

You can find a wide variety of scents at many retail outlets, but your best bet in finding great, long-lasting scents is to go to places such as Sephora, Ulta, or retail giants such as Sachs Fifth Avenue or Macy's. It must be stated up front that, more often than not, a higher end cologne or perfume will indeed cost a pretty penny. It won't be cheap, and you have to shell out a large amount of cash for Chanel, Dior, Burberry, or John Varvatos. But the good thing is, these scents will last you quite a long time. Cheaper cologne and perfume manufacturers do—for lack of a better term—cut their fragrances with water and other low-end material. The preferred, higher-end scent makers do not. So you are paying for quality, and you're paying a decent amount for it, but you're also purchasing something that's going to last you a good number of months, if not years. With the better fragrances, you only have to use just a little bit for it to last throughout the day. This can result in keeping a bottle of your favorite stuff for many months if not many years.

So, how do you pick what perfume or cologne to buy? Simple. Plan a day where you and your loved one can head out to one of the aforementioned stores or another perfume vendor, and start checking out the scents! Find the ones that you love, that drive you crazy, that put a smile on your face, and try them out. Remember, smell the perfume's scent first before putting it on. There will more than likely be little pieces of cardstock paper that you can spray the fragrance onto.

Do not put on scent after scent. You'll run the risk of tainting the original scent with a new one. You don't want that. Many fine retailers will usually have a small container filled with coffee beans. This acts as an olfactory pallet cleanser. Think of it as a glass of water after drinking a shot of bourbon, or a sliver of ginger after eating a few pieces of sushi. Pick a fragrance, smell it, and then take a hearty whiff of the coffee bean container. When you move on to the next perfume or cologne, your sense of smell will be clean and ready to experience the next one.

Once you've found two or three scents that you're really into, dab a little on your wrists, or on your neck. If it comes in a spray bottle (which most scents do), spray just a touch of perfume on those areas. You don't want to douse yourself, but you also don't want to run the risk of not putting enough on. Remember, it's not just the scent in the bottle. It's also your natural pheromones. You have to know how both the perfume or cologne and your natural body scent work together. Sometimes what's in a bottle can smell great, but after you put it on and leave it on for a little while, the smell isn't as appealing. And sometimes the reverse is true as well. Sometimes the scent in the bottle might not be exactly what appeals to you, but you put it on, and your significant other tells you that you've never smelled better!

It's trial and error, really. You just have to hunt down what you like and keep your eyes (and nostrils) open. And don't forget, there are people who work in those stores, who are trained to help you with these kinds of things. Talk with them, and ask them about what their favorite perfumes or colognes are. Have them tell you a little about what they've found to be some of the better, longer lasting scents. In the end, you'll get a great fragrance, they make a sale, and your partner gets to experience a new you through one of his or her five senses. It's a win-win-win situation for everyone involved!

Granted, to most guys and to some women, the idea of spending a number of hours in a store checking out row after row and shelf after shelf of bottles of scents may not seem like the best way to spend a morning or afternoon. But remember, this is all about setting yourself and the both of you up for a night (and many nights thereafter) of passion! So, in the grand scheme of things, a few hours in a store is nothing in comparison to having a thousand-and-one orgasms.

And when we're talking about scent and pleasant smelling additions to our person, we don't just use colognes or perfumes, soaps, deodorants, shampoos and body washes play a part as well. These items can be a great way to enhance your natural scent and get your partner's senses reeling, and they can interlock with those perfumes and colognes to give a person's body an overall pleasant appeal. A good thing to do is to find the aforementioned items that have a similar or adds a complimentary scent to the perfume or cologne of your choice. For instance, if a guy chooses to wear cologne that has a scented mixture of tobacco and vanilla, then they should seek out a body wash or soap that has those scents within. If a woman chooses to wear a floral scent perfume, then the body wash should be similar.

And when we're speaking of scent, it's not just what we put on that makes us more attractive to our loved one, it can be what we do with the room we're in. Scented candles or oils can enhance the eroticism level. A nice smelling home is a great way to get a couple in the mood. Vātsyāyana mentions in a number of passages in the Kama Sutra of a 'Chamber of Love,' or 'Love Chamber' (depending on the translation) which is accented to a greater extent by flowers, oils, and incense. Whatever smells you and your partner enjoy, whether it be juniper, citric, lilac, sandalwood, or patchouli, get a couple of candles, oil burners, or incense sticks, and let them fill the room or home.

Sight

It is certain that it goes without saying (but we'll say it anyway), that a woman in gorgeous lingerie is one of the most erotic, sexy, and beautiful things that a man will ever lay his eyes on. And it's almost an accepted fact that a man who wears a suit somehow becomes much more attractive. These bits of clothing, these things that we drape upon our bodies, they're almost like superhero costumes! We go from a mild-mannered working stiff to a sexy beast just with the simple act of putting on a tie, or a little see-through negligee. Really, it's amazing.

Whether it is a power suit, or something from Victoria's Secret, or a little costume you can order online, you should have the initiative to get whatever your partner likes onto your body... and then off your body as quickly as possible if the mood is right!

Before we go any further, let's eradicate one common misconception about men and women. The commonly held myth is that men are way more visual than women when it comes to sexual arousal. While it is true that men probably place visual stimulation at the top of their list, (if they were creating such a list in the first place) women are visual as well. The difference is, as many studies have shown over the past number of years, is that men tend to take the visual stimuli and want to act on that desire right away. Women, on the other hand, can take in that stimuli and ruminate on it, let it linger, let it swell up inside their thoughts.

As crass as it might sound, men see a nice pair of legs or breasts, and automatically their brains are hardwired into giving in to almost immediate orgasm. Women see a pair of biceps or a nice butt and want to take a mental snapshot of it and examine it in their heads over and over and over again.

But whatever the case, or whatever the studies tell us, we have to get rid of that old, dusty, rusted, broken down idea that it's only guys who like looking at bodies. Women love it too. So, let's give 'em both what they want!

The quickest way to do this is to find out what your significant other likes to see you wearing (besides nothing). Guys, if your partner loves seeing you in that aforementioned suit, then find almost any excuse you can to put one on. Ladies, if your lover loves seeing you clad in a nightie, or a silk robe, or whatever, then buy two of whatever it is that they like. And maybe ask a few questions. Probe them. Ask for details. It might turn out that your hubby has a thing for a French maid's outfit. Or your wife might have a thing for silk boxers. We might be getting to the point where we sound like a broken record, but as we stated, right at the beginning of the book, communication is key.

Sound

We mentioned it earlier in this book, but talking dirty can be a great way to get your partner in the mood and keep them in the mood. But in the aspect of making yourself more and more attractive to your partner, it's not just what you say, it's how you say it.

Work on your voice. Get your 'sexy' going with your vocal cords. Ladies, work on your phone sex operator voice. Guys, get your timbre, low and commanding. For some of us, just hearing a hot voice is more than enough to set the right tone.

Believing

What is it about Kid Rock? What about Mick Jagger back in the day? What in the hell is it about Gene Simmons? He'll be the first to tell you that he's slept with thousands of women. But he'll also be the first to tell you that he's not the most attractive guy in the world. What about some politicians or world leaders who aren't the male model types but yet have their share of groupies as well? And what is it about a woman, say an actress or female comedian, who might not fit the atypical, 'good looking' stereotype but is for some unknowable reason just plain sexy?

Here's the secret: it's confidence.

Beyond the scent, beyond the visual, beyond the auditory, there is one final piece of the attractiveness puzzle, and it's something that you can't buy, manufacture, or pluck out of thin air. You have to believe that you are stunning. You have to believe that you have that swagger. You have to believe that you are a god or goddess amongst mere mortals.

So... Kid Rock? Ever see the guy on stage? You may not like the music, in fact, you may despise it, but there's no denying that the man can work a stage. And speaking of working a stage... Jagger? Seriously, you would be hard-pressed to come up with a better front man for a rock band. Even in his seventh decade of life, Mick moves with the ability and effortlessness of someone half, or one-third, his age! Gene Simmons? You know the old KISS tagline right? "You wanted the best, you got the best!" Simmons is there to give you the best show you'll ever see in your life, and he'll put one-hundred-thousand percent into it. These things are want comes from swagger, and whatever you may think of these guys on a personal, moral, or sexual level, the facts speak for themselves. Their charisma, their charm, and their belief in themselves have earned them millions of fans the world over, and, simply put, countless groupies willing to do almost anything to please them.

Again, charisma is an undefinable thing. It's not tangible. You can't put it in a bottle and sell it at a store. If you could, whatever company that figured out how to do so would be making cash hand over fist.

As another — shall we say — well laid person from the rock and roll world, Lemmy Kilmister (of the band Motörhead, who claimed on a number of occasions to have slept with over a thousand women, may he rest in peace) once said, "The people with the best charisma don't even know they have it." But if we can just take all of the tips and ideas in this book and utilize them over and over again, it won't be too long before our partners start to see us as the main objects of their fantasies.

Chapter 5: Keep It Up

Throughout this book, we've discussed open and honest communication between sexual partners, flirtation, foreplay, sex, sexual positions, kinks, fetishes, and general sexual interests. But we've saved the most important part of any sexual relationship until the very end. This is our climax if you'll allow us a coy turn of phrase.

Here's the thing, it's not only important to have a good sexual relationship with your partner, to speak openly about what you're interested in, what you want to try, what you need from them, and what you would like to experience together, but it's even more important to keep trying and doing these things again and again and again. Find what you like, do that thing, and keep exploring. Don't settle. Don't become stilted. Don't let the grass grow under your feet. Shake the dust off and keep on going.

As we've said before, a tiny little spark can start the greatest fire, but as is the case with all fires, you have to keep watch over them. You have to keep adding to it, stoking it, fanning it, letting it breathe, giving it air, and letting it flourish. Without continuous attention and a deft sense of vigilance, the fire can die, sometimes very slowly, sometimes very quickly, and there's nothing worse in a relationship, sexual or otherwise, than to feel that cold, cold distance between you and the one you so love, need, want, and desire in your life.

Another aspect of keeping the flame of your love burning is to not allow the responsibility of being the keeper of the flame to fall squarely on the shoulders of just one person. Both people involved in the relationship need to chip in and do their part to continue building that fire. It cannot, and should not, be the job of the woman in the relationship to always come up with ideas to build up romance. It shouldn't be up to the husband to do the lion's share of the talking when he wants to express new things that he wants to try in the bedroom. If there are two (or, let's face it, in some cases, more) people in a romantic partnership, there isn't any room whatsoever for a pilot and co-pilot, a lead singer and a backup singer, a lead actor and supporting actor. It's all even, it's all equal, and the responsibilities that come along with being equals also fall into the realm of the bedroom. In other words, you're both in this together, so act like it.

In the introduction of this text, we also spoke about using it as sort of a stepping stone towards reading the actual Kama Sutra. Since you're at the end of this book, you should consider moving on and reading Vātsyāyana's tome. However, you should also take caution once you decide to do so. Vātsyāyana not only spoke at length about the pleasures that two people could have, but also about setting a proper mood for lovemaking, paying attention to a woman's needs, and things of that nature, but he also does tend to dip his toe, and in some cases, dwell too long in areas such as giving advice on how to seduce another man's wife, the great business aspect of being a pimp in charge of prostitutes, and, basically, how a man can trick a woman into sleeping with him.

Taken in its historical context, the Kama Sutra is, for all purposes, a rather forward-thinking book. The very idea that a Hindu text, written supposedly about 2,000 years ago, that even mentions the idea of giving a woman sexual gratification, and giving advice and instruction on how to make an equal partnership in a married couple's home life, is frankly astonishing. Exploring the G-spot, or foreplay, or the pleasures of oral sex between both sexes, are concepts that would not even be committed to texts until well into the 19th or 20th century, and are still, to this day, banned in some places, and undoubtedly looked down upon in others. But, as stated, there are certain cases in the overall text that could be seen as rather misogynistic and somewhat hateful towards women. Please keep this in mind before picking up a copy of the Kama Sutra, but also keep in mind that the tome, for its few faults, it's still well worth the read.

Also, as much as possible, please try to find the most recent translation. Many people in the English-speaking world still read the Sir Richard Francis Burton translation. Burton was a British explorer and translator of two highly popular texts which were made available to the people of Britain, Canada, Ireland, and the United States in the late 1800s, The Arabian Nights and the Kama Sutra. Although technically, Burton didn't fully translate the Kama Sutra on his own, (fellow Englishman Forster Fitzgerald Arbuthnot helped tremendously with translating it) he has long been considered the main source of getting the tome into the hands of the native English speakers. However, a book entitled Redeeming the Kamasutra by Wendy Doniger published in 2016 cites mistranslations, misconceptions, and failures in verbiage and syntax in the Burton/Arbuthnot text. Doniger does give credit where it's due, but her account of the sometimes mind-boggling ways the original translation came about makes for an insightful and oftentimes, a hilarious read.

And, finally, we can't stress this enough, take what you've learned here, what you will learn if you decide to read the Kama Sutra in its entirety, and put your own spin on these concepts! In other words, write your own new chapters of the Kama Sutra! Making these ideas all your own can only enhance the relationship that you have with your partner. Again, this is all about you and your loved one. Learn! Grow! Explore! Invent! Improvise! Be one with one another! Be at peace! Be in love! Release your lust! Be involved! And don't ever, ever lose that single, solitary spark.

There are many things worth fighting and dying for in this world, and love is the number one thing. Some days the battle can be tense, long, drawn out, and make you feel like you're at your wit's end. But always bear in mind that without love, we're barely human. Again, again, again, love is always worth it. And having that connection with another person and strengthening that connection by any means necessary and available to ourselves makes one feel alive, electric, and at one with the universe. If there's something you should have garnered from the tips, ideas, and statements from this text, it's that love is valuable and please, always remember that.

And of course, don't forget to have lots and lots of great sex! Peace, love, and respect to all of you.

Conclusion

Thank you for making it through to the end of this book. Let's hope it was informative, entertaining, uplifting, insightful, and that the eBook was able to provide you with all of the tools you need to achieve your goals in your sex life, personal relationship, and interaction with your loved one.

If you did find this book useful in any way, shape, or form, leaving a review on Amazon is always appreciated! And we would also be thankful if you recommend this book to anyone you know that may find what it has to offer to their liking. Don't be afraid to spread the word!

Thank you again for your purchase! So long, and happy reading!

Kama Sutra Sex Positions

The Ultimate Guide on Kama Sutra with 121+ Sex Positions for Exploding your Sex Life, Increase Intimacy, Increase Libido and Improve Your Relationship with your Partner.

Lana Fox

contained within this document, including, but not limited to, — errors, omissions, or inaccuracies.

Contents

Chapter 1: Kama Sutra 110

Chapter 2: Flirting and Courtship 148

Chapter 3: Intimacy 162

Chapter 4: Foreplay 181

Chapter 5: Sex Positions 195

Conclusion.. 342

Chapter 1: Kama Sutra

Did you know the Kama Sutra was written by a celibate scholar? Or that the Kama Sutra revolves around a man's pleasure? Or that only about 20% of the book is about sexual positioning? It's interesting that most people know about Kama Sutra and yet they don't really know what it is about.

After being with the same partner for a number of years, many couples are desperately curious about how to spice up their sex life. Stuck for options, they secretly tiptoe down the "sex" section of the bookstore to get a peek at the Kama Sutra nudie pictures and acrobatic sexual positions. Titillated, they buy the book only to have it sit untouched and lonesome in their nightstand drawer forevermore.

Unfortunately, they failed to understand that Kama Sutra is not a sex-quick-fix; rather, it's a comprehensive way of looking at their sexuality. As such, it has remained under its mystical Eastern shroud since it first hit pop-culture in the early 1980s.

Truthfully, the Kama Sutra isn't all that complicated and it's a great way for couples to keep their sex fun and fresh over the long term.

So what is Kama Sutra? It was meant as a pillow book. Whereas our Western culture believed in not talking about sex and leaving kids ignorant until their wedding day, Eastern culture had the opposite viewpoint. When a young person became engaged, they were given a "pillow book", which was their technical guide on how to have sex. Vatsyayana happened to create the world's most famous pillow book.

Tradition believes Vatsyayana was a celibate scholar who lived sometime around 4th century AD. He did not write the Kama Sutra per se; rather, he was a compiler and editor of all the information that existed during the very rich Gupta period. Interestingly, Vatsyayana believed that sex itself was not wrong, but doing it frivolously was sinful.

Therefore, "Kama" literally means desire and "Sutra" signifies a thread or a thread of discourses. While most of us believe the Kama Sutra is all about sexual positions, 80% of the book gives insights on how to make love a divine union, how to act like a responsible citizen, how to handle your household, etc. It's a discourse or a marriage manual to troubleshoot all the sticky points a young man or young woman will face in their pending marriage. Brilliant, really.

And then there are the infamous 64 positions which has launched hundreds (maybe thousands) of books, videos and websites. Vatsyayana believed there were eight ways to make love, multiplied by eight positions. A veritable smorgasbord.

What many people don't realize is that the Kama Sutra's focus is to give the man the maximum amount of sexual pleasure. Eastern culture believed that, in order for the man to get the maximum amount of gratification, he first had to bring the woman to full arousal. Why? The more sexual energy she had, the more likely her energy would cross over to give him a bigger, better orgasm.

What does that translate to? Our quickly-becomes-boring Western get-on, get-in, get-off type of sex cannot begin to rival Kama Sutra's sex because it is about the entire sexual experience.

Kama Sutra sex has a beginning, middle and end-instead of just focusing on the middle like Westerns do. First, the Kama Sutra gives instructions on how to prepare yourself and your environment for lovemaking. It then talks about multiple ways to have foreplay in order to "energize" the woman (yeah!). It then shows many different options for positions. The possible combinations are endless, enabling you to mix-up sex each and every time.

You may be asking, "If Kama Sutra is so great, why aren't more people jumping on the band wagon?" Well, if you go totally authentic and read Richard Burton's original translated version of Vatsyayana's work, it is deathly boring. Did I mention complicated? He talks about yonis and bulls and other euphemisms that are unfamiliar to our Western sensibilities. It's intimidating and off-putting for the average couple.

Luckily, Anne Hooper came out with Kama Sutra for 21st Century Lovers. It's the best version I've seen on the store shelf because it is written in understandable language and the photos are superb. Or if you want to go more authentic, Deepak Chopra is trying to cash in on his name with his beautiful version of Kama Sutra.

If you've done the math, yes Kama Sutra takes more bedroom work. Time starved couples look at it, roll their eyes and say, "No thanks." Please remember though, good sex gives you and your relationship a much-needed injection of energy. The ten or fifteen minutes of extra time will take your sex from blah to bravo.

There is profound spiritual energy in love and intimacy. Tantric (or Transformative) yoga is a spiritual system, if you will, and in Tantric teachings, sexual love is a sacrament, and Tantra's goals are more exalted and broader in scope than simply to accomplish proficiency in sex. The ultimate goal is spiritual union with the cosmic consciousness, God, or whatever your particular words are for a higher power. Tantra can both elevate and deepen a couple's relationship. Think of it as the art of conscious loving. Tomes have been written on it and it's certainly worthy of deeper exploration.

For Dr. Johanina Wikoff, noted psychologist and Tantric instructor, the door to Tantra that she had been searching for opened when a book literally fell from a bookshelf and landed at her feet. The book was "Tantra, Spirituality and Sex," by Osho Rajneesh. She picked it up and sat down to read it on the spot. She recalls, "It was exactly what I had been looking for. It was about reverence, it was about honoring, and about lovemaking as a meditation and a sacrament, a celebration and liberation. It won me over and I began reading every thing that I could."

Says Wikoff earnestly, "The most important thing in lovemaking, the thing that makes for great sex, and even good sex, is the ability to be present, to be present in your body, to be present to your partner, to their touch, the way they smell, the way they feel, aware of everything about them. To feel and fully experience the sensations of the moment. Being present is very simple. It is attention and breath. If you take a deep breath, you can't be in the past, or worrying about the things that might happen tomorrow. When you are paying attention to the breath and to the body, you are present, you are right there. That is what I do with people; I teach them how to be present to their experiences."

Tantra, as Wikoff discovered, has informed and inspired generations in the art of lovemaking and conjugal skills. This controversial body of wisdom includes art, music, poetry, science, philosophy and, to a lesser degree, the martial arts. It appeared in India sometime around the 8th century and flourished there for more than 400 years, during which time it spread into Tibet and eventually China and Japan. As Tantric teachings radiated throughout the East, they inspired new schools of intimacy such as the Tibetan Arts of Love, the Japanese Pillow Book, Taoism, and the fabled Kama Sutra in India. All of these children of Tantra have one thing in common: a reverence for the spirit of ecstasy.

Wikoff's search had begun several years earlier when she walked away from the soul-draining demands of her advertising career in order to create a more rewarding, sustainable life. She headed for the peace and unhurried pace of the Northern California mountains. After settling in, she put her energy into starting a community school for children and recalls, "Once I got there, built a house, and started working with the kids, I realized that I needed something to keep me from going crazy without the distraction of the world. It occurred to me that meditation would be a very good and natural thing to do. So I began meditating and was drawn to the teachings of a man named Chogyam Trungpa Rinpoche."

Trungpa, a Tibetan Buddhist, was one of the people most responsible for popularizing Buddhism in America and who eventually founded the renowned Naropa School in Boulder, Colorado. Wikoff began to study Trungpa's work in earnest and was thrilled when he opened a meditation center nearby. "It was through his teaching that I eventually became aware of Tantra," she remembers. "So I began asking questions and kept hearing references to this little known left-hand path that has to do with sexuality. When I would ask why we were not studying this, I was told, 'It's very dangerous. You must study for a very long time.'"

She did. And although the trail of her studies would turn out to be a winding one, a common thread guided her -- her desire to understand the breath and the role that it can play in accessing and understanding emotions.

"My awareness of the importance of breathing developed while we were snowed in one winter," she recalls. "I was suffering from a bronchial asthma attack and spent two weeks treating myself with herbs and struggling from one breath to the next. During that time I noticed that emotions started coming up, memories began coming up, and I was aware of every thought in my mind. I recognized that it was a powerful gateway, a vehicle for knowing myself and understanding where I was cut off from my feelings. I decided that when I recovered, I was going to learn all I could about the breath."

She started with yoga, herbs, and meditation techniques, and then eventually discovered Reichian therapy and bioenergetics. "Once I got to the Reichian therapies I had the big 'aha!'" she exclaims. "Oh, I see now! When we hold emotions in the body we hold our breath! When we are afraid, what do we do? We hold our breath. When we are angry or in shock, we hold our breath. Once I recognized that connection I continued to explore, and one teacher led to another. I eventually synthesized what I do now, what I know now, which is specializing in relationships and sexuality."

As Dr. Wikoff discovered, however, this kind of keen breath awareness in Tantra can unearth emotional issues and memories that have been buried for years. People may find that they are angry with their partner, or that they have recollections of unpleasant experiences or abuse. If these issues arise, they must be worked through and resolved. But the ability of this intimate awareness to remove the barriers to communication and honesty is what makes it so powerful and compelling. When you achieve this, when you are present, aware, and breathing, the body relaxes and becomes more receptive. At that point the energy that is generated during lovemaking can expand and flow through your whole body. This is the foundation of all Tantric techniques.

"Sexuality is such a powerful force," she continues. "It brings everything to the surface. In our culture we have so much addiction. One could use Tantra as an excuse to indulge those addictions. This is why it is such a dangerous path, and why it requires years of experience to master. You have to be attentive and able to recognize when you are conscious and respectful, and when you are losing yourself and becoming indulgent. Tantra teaches us that if we are mindful and present, we can indulge in our passions and desires without letting them control us. Knowing yourself and being aware is the way of Tantra."

Tantra will likely remain a source of controversy, but not for Wikoff. When she stepped in to that Northern California bookstore and began the journey down the "left hand" path, she found the new life she had been seeking; a life that exchanged the buzz and bustle of the boardroom for awareness, presence and desire. With it came the opportunity for her to not only find personal fulfillment, but to teach a new generation of seekers how to breathe deeply, embrace life, and create more passion and love in their lives.

Kama Sutra - All The Goals Of The Kama Sutra

The Kama Sutra was written by Mallanaga Vatsyayana in ancient Sanskrit. It was written in accordance with the purusharthas of Indian tradition as its basis. These purusharthas are commonly referred to as the four Main goals of life. By ancient Hindu tradition, these goals were key to escaping the cycle of reincarnation, or being reborn in different castes and states according to the actions of a previous lifetime. These goals were Dharma, Artha, Kama and Moksha. The first three goals, Dharma, Artha and Kama are portions of everday existence whereas Moksha was the highest goal achieved by reaching the three earthly goals. The achievement of the goal, Moksha, meant that one would be released from the cycle of death and rebirth.

According to Vatsyayana, as translated by Sir Richard Francis Burton, "Dharma is better than Artha, and Artha is better than Kama. But Artha should always be first practised by the king for the livelihood of men is to be obtained from it only. Again, Kama being the occupation of public women, they should prefer it to the other two, and these are exceptions to the general rule." (Kama Sutra 1.2.14) Thus it can be seen that each of the goals was ranked according to its own value in the scheme of things.

Dharma - Virtuous Living

The first goal is Dharma or Virtuous Living. This goal implied leading a life of moral values and doing good works. The individual seeking to achieve Dharma would seek to avoid ill will and injury to others. In some traditions, the pursuit of Dharma was even extended to animal and insect life to the point that a man was not allowed to kill an insect. While many people would not consider the Kama Sutra to be a particularly moral text, there is a very high placement given to Dharma or Virtuous Living. Dharma is considered such a high goal that whenever two motives conflict, Dharma is always the path to be followed.

Artha - Material Prosperity

The second goal of life, according to Vatsyayana and his Kama Sutra, was the pursuit of Artha or Material Prosperity. This goal made certain that a man's household was well provided for. As long as a man's living did not interfere with his Virtue, it was considered to be a distinguishing point to be gainfully employed. The proper Hindu gentleman worked very hard to make certain that the goal of Artha was satisfied by making a good life for him and his househeld.

Kama - Aesthetic And Erotic Pleasure

Kama or Aesthetic and Erotic Pleasure is the third goal of life according to the Kama Sutra. This goal also lends it's name to the title of the text as Vatsyayana peened the ancient Sanskrit tome as a guide to putting the pursuit of Kama in its proper place. Kama is the lowest of the three motives and was considered "the occupation of public women" or prostitutes. Kama was the pursuit of physical pleasure and had it's proper place in the life of a Hindu gentleman. This motive has become the focal point for many individuals in their definition of the Kama Sutra even though the goal of the text was to put Karma in it's proper place as the lowest of the three motives.

For the those looking for spiritual enlightenment along the Hindu path to Moksha or for those who seek a simple way of putting life into perspective, Vatsyayana's Kama Sutra has much to offer in the way of teaching.

The Content Of The Kama Sutra

The Kama Sutra written by Vatsyayana consisted of seven sections further divided into thirty-six chapters. We will discuss each of these sections to glean the details of what Vatsyayana was trying to convey in the Kama Sutra and the importance he placed on specific subjects.

Section One - Introductory

The first section of the Kama Sutra consisted of five chapters explaining the contents of the manuscript, the three major aims and priorities of life according to the Hindu belief system of the day, the acquisition of knowledge, suitable conduct for the well-bred townsman and various reflections on intermediaries who assist the lover in his enterprises.

Section Two- On Sexual Union

The second section of the Kama Sutra consisted of ten chapters on the stimulation of desire, various forms of embraces, caressing and kisses, marking a partner with the use of the finger nails, biting and marking a partner using the teeth, on positions of copulation, explanations of sexual practices such as slapping with the hand and moaning that accompanied the practice, evidence of virile behavior in women, superior coitus and oral sex practices, along with preludes and conclusions to the game of love. There are 64 types of sexual acts described in this section which has become the part of the Kama Sutra for which the book is most widely known.

Section Three - About The Acquisition Of A Wife

Section three of the Kama Sutra consists of Five chapters on the forms of marriage, how to relax and obtain the girl, how to manage alone when a suitable wife cannot be found and the union by marriage.

Section Four- About A Wife

Section four consist of counsel to the various types of wives a Hindu gentleman may have had. There are two chapters dealing with the conduct of the wives. The section of the Kama Sutra yields advice to the solitary wife in how she should conduct herself. This section of the Kama Sutra also explained the conduct of the chief wife and other wives in a household with multiple wives and concubines.

Section Five - About The Wives Of Other People

This section of the Kama Sutra consisted of six chapters on behavior of women and men. It included advice on the methods of seducing another mans wife, including encounters for getting acquainted, examination of sentiments, the tasks and advantages of go-betweens, the king's pleasures such as his harem and ways the brave could circumvent security measures and enjoy those pleasures themselves, as well as the proper behavior of a Hindu gentleman in the gynoecium or womens apartments.

Section Six - About Courtesans

Section Six of the Kama Sutra consisted of six chapters on making the best use of the advice of the assistants on choosing lovers, the search for a steady lover, the courtesans skill set and ways of making money, how best to renew friendship with a former lover, creating occasional profits and dealing with profits and losses associated with being a courtesan.

Section Seven - On The Means Of Attracting Others To One's Self

The two chapters of section seven of the Kama Sutra deal mainly with thoughts on improving physical attractiveness to others and arousing a weakened or failing sexual power.

Male And Female Enhancement of The Kama Sutra

Vatsyayana freely admitted that even the god of love can sometimes have a poor aim. When he does, strange unions form as can be understood by the following quote from the Kama Sutra: "Sometimes Kama, absent-minded, throws his arrow haphazardly. Thus one sees strange couples assembling. A man and a woman who should not have been brought together. They attract criticism, mockery and yet, 'badly-matched' love defies time! This hare-man, thin and graceful, adores his elephant wife, as powerful as a giant.

Their tastes, their preoccupations, their bodies, are discordant. But they adore each other! And, in the games of love, their harmony is perfect. The hare-man knows all the subtle caresses that arouse his wife. Making use of Apadravyas, he increases the size of his frail lingam. There are all kinds of them in the pleasure room: gold armband, precious wood tube, ivory bracelet. They choose them according to how their lovemaking progresses."

We have all met couples that just don't appear to be well suited for each other and yet they seem to thrive on the others company. Just as the couple mentioned in the Kama Sutra, we find very thin men with much larger women or small statured ladies in love with men who appear to be mountains. It isn't a new fad by any means. What advice did the Kama Sutra offer these couples to make their sexual encounters more pleasurable for both parties?

Ancient Male Enhancement Secrets Of The Kama Sutra

Aside from the above recommendation of supplying a less than adequate lover with attachments to increase length and girth, the Kama Sutra offered another bit of advice. This came in the form of a recipe for an ancient form of male enhancement. Let's take a look at this ancient secret in the words of the Kama Sutra itself.
"First rub your lingam with wasp stings and massage it with sweet oil. When it swells, let it dangle for ten nights through a hole in your bed, going to sleep each night on your stomach.
After this period use a cool ointment to remove the pain and swelling. By this method men of insatiable sexual appetite, manage to keep their lingam enlarged throughout their lives."
That prescription makes those Apradavya's, or sexual accessories mentioned above, look like a walk in the park. I don't know about you, but, personally, I would rather be laughed at by every woman I ever met than try that particular cure.

Ointments For Female Enhancement From The Kama Sutra

It seems that while Vatsyayana's advice may have been a bit masochistic for the men, he was a little easier on the ladies. In the Kama Sutra, he described two different ointments with different purposes.

For the ladies who were of a size that was a bit too large for their man to accommodate them, the Kama Sutra provided the following insights: "By applying an ointment made from crushed Barleria leaves to her yoni, the elephant woman can spend at least one night discovering the delights of being a doe."

If she happened to over do the effect or was just to small to accommodate a larger male to begin with he had a different ointment. He went on to say, "Likewise the doe can use honey mixed with powdered roots of Lotus, Madder, Sal (tree of aromatic gum), the Blue Lotus and the Mongoose plant to accommodate a stallion for one night.

Growing Closer With The Embracing Positions Of The Kama Sutra

The Kama Sutra of Vatsyayana was intended as a lesson in proper decorum and relationships between Hindu couples of its time. Just as their modern counterparts, ancient couples sought after a deeper level of intimacy with each other and a feeling of closeness. It penned the Kama Sutra in hopes of helping his peers to achieve the goals of life, including the goal of Sutra, and to put these goals in proper prospective. One of the recommended forms in the Kama Sutra was the positions of Embracing as they provided for a special closeness.

Why Is Embracing Important?

It is quite amazing how much feeling can be communicated by an embrace or hug. As children, we are comforted in times of pain or sickness by a mothers loving arms. As we grow older, we still seek out that close bond with others as way to feel loved and appreciated. With an embrace, we can express condolence, affection, protection or comfort. In the Kama Sutra, Vatsyayana recognized the importance that an embrace could hold in a relationship between lovers. He realized that the simple act of embracing could convey the deep emotions and security that the mates provided for each other and a feeling of connecting of their souls. With these thoughts in mind, he recommended the Embracing positions of the Kama Sutra.

What Are The Embracing Positions Of The Kama Sutra?

Vatsyayana related a variety of embracing positions in the Kama Sutra with two varieties for standing embrace being the The Twining of the Creeper which the Kama Sutra describes as, "When a woman, clinging to a man as a creeper twines round a tree, bends his head down to hers with the desire of kissing him and slightly makes the sound of sut sut, embraces him, and looks lovingly towards him." and the Climbing of a Tree which they explained as being, "When a woman, having placed one of her feet on the foot of her lover, and the other on one of his thighs, passes one of her arms round his back, and the other on his shoulders, makes slightly the sounds of singing and cooing, and wishes, as it were, to climb up him in order to have a kiss."

The Kama Sutra goes on to relate several embracing positions to be applied at the time of sexual union. These were known as The Mixture of Sesamum Seed with Rice and The Mixture of Milk and Water. Both of these positions were intended to induce closeness and a sense of melting two bodies into one.

Vatsyayana's Kama Sutra went on to describe four lesser embraces as well that involved more specific areas of the body rather than the complete embraces mentioned above. These four embraces are conveyed to us as The Embrace of the Thighs, The Embrace of the Jaghana (or. the part of the body from the navel downwards to the thighs), The Embrace of the Breasts and The Embrace of the Forehead.

A Brief Look At The Kama Sutra

The ancient Sanskrit text of the Kamasutram, more commonly known in western culture as the Kama Sutra, was originally written by Mallanaga Vatsyayana and is believed to be a master work on the ways of Love in all its forms. The Kama Sutra is just one, though the most notable, of a larger collection of ancient Indian texts known as the Kama Shastra or Discipline of Kama.

These texts were originally of a religious nature and common theology holds that the collection was handed down to mankind by Shiva's doorkeeper, Nandi the sacred bull, after hearing the god, Shiva and Parvati, his wife having relations. The session so inspired the sacred bull to make utterance which was later recorded and passed down to mankind for their benefit. It is believed that the present form of the Kama Sutra is a compendium that was gathered at some point in the second century CE.

What is the Kama Sutra?

Etmylogically speaking, Kama Sutra can be broken down into two Sanskrit words; the first being Kama, which is a reference to the Hindu god of Love, using the same name. In common language, it conveyed the ideas of desire, wish, intention, pleasure and love, especially in a sexual connotation. In chapter two of Richard Burton's translation of the text, Kama is translated as "the enjoyment of appropriate objects by the five senses of hearing, feeling, seeing, tasting and smelling, assisted by the mind together with the soul. The ingredient in this is a peculiar contact between the organ of sense and its object, and the consciousness of pleasure which arises from that contact is called Kama."

The second word, Sutra refers to a discourse delivered on a set of concise rules. Thus Sutra has the connotation of a technical study or manual. Thus, the Sutra was intended to educate the reader in the field of it's particular study.

Taken together, the words Kama Sutra imply a technical text on the aspects of properly enjoying the stimulation of the five senses and the demonstration of Love. Unfortunately, the simple wording of the title has led to many misconceptions regarding the text and it is to be noted that the Kama Sutra is nether a sex manual or a sacred religious text, though it does incorporate both aspects into its writing. While the text is explicit in details of a sexual nature and also intones highly religious themes, it was intended to put Kama in to context with the other two aims of ancient Hindu life, Dharma and Artha. This is evidenced by Vatsyayana's opening discussion of these three aims at the beginning of the text.

These three terms are described as relating to Virtue (Dharma), Material Prosperity (Artha) and Pleasure (Kama) and they were to be pursued in that order. The first quality almost always took precedence over the secondary when two of these pursuits were at odds, though there were a few exceptions to this rule. Thus being virtuous was to be sought more than wealth but pleasure would fall secondary to the pursuit of material gain in the Hindu way of life. The Kama Sutra was intended as a guide to show how to properly achieve all three goals and their proper places so as to achieve Moksha, the liberation from the cycle of reincarnation.

The Moral Repercussions Of The Kama Sutra

At the time Vatsyayana penned the words of the Kama Sutra, he had no idea what he was beginning. He and his contemporaries were highly educated, religious men of the Hindu faith. The work that Vatsyayana put onto parchment was not intended as a corrupting influence but was more the advice of one who had traveled a path and wanted to share the knowledge of the journey. Even though, Vatsyayana refers to "public women" or prostitutes, explaining the differences between them and their uses, and coaches his male students on the proper way to seduce a married woman while admitting that relations with another mans mate are to be avoided, he was a fairly moral man for the society of his time. If he and his contemporaries could see the later works of today, they might question our own moral fiber.

What Did Vatsyayana Start?

Vatsyayana published the Kama Sutra as a way of sharing his knowledge but to some societies this knowledge would seem ill gained. He spoke of the use of consorts, both male and female, and of various forms of sexual intercourse. These positions came as quite a shock to Victorian era English men and women when Sir Richard Burton published the first English translation of the work. While it outwardly brought fainting, shuddering and a conflagration, in private people were titillated by the work and it began to eat at the back of their minds just how some of those positions worked and whether that male enhancement recipe that called for the stings of a wasp really did work permanently. Burton, himself having three Indian mistresses, was quoted to say,"We British never knew of this kind of love-making. Had we known, we would not have ruined the lives of so many British virgins." This comment was made after his visit to a prostitute of the day. While folks claimed an aversion to the subject matter, they were privately drawn to it and the morals of the society began a subtle change.

As the secrets of the Kama Sutra slowly leaked out, the common man thought to himself that this or that new idea sounded quite interesting. For a time period when the missionary position was the only church sanctioned union, some of the ideas of the Kama Sutra must have sounded very intriguing. Now and then a recipient of the Kama Sutra's knowledge would decide to give something a try and come back with a sore back or a pulled tendon but with each torn ligament there was also a tear in the morals of the society.

How Far Did This Influence Reach?

The influence of the Kama Sutra did not stop with the English countryside. Far from it, the influence has spread to nearly all parts of the world and has become even more pervasive as the quality of communication has increased. With the Internet and the eased restrictions on the publications of printed material;s, the Kama Sutra finds a larger following all the time. Unfortunately, many people have forgotten Vatsyayna's original goal for the Kama Sutra which was to put sex and its pleasures in their proper perspective. Society has become very promiscuous and quick to go for what feels good to the individual. Thus we find a moral breakdown unparalleled by any other time in history.

Kama Sutra - The Proper Application

When Vatsyayana first penned the Kama Sutra, he had a few important things in mind. He wanted to teach proper Hindu gentlemen of his time the lessons about the major goals in life and how these goals were to be obtained. One of those goals was Sutra, or pleasure derived from experiences. Though the term Sutra could mean pleasure from other than erotic or sexual stimulus, the Kama Sutra has come to be synonymous with sexually learned and those who have studied it find themselves sought after as sexual partners.

While the sexual aspect of the Kama Sutra alone is very educational, the further development of attached emotions and philosophy was also important to Vatsyayana when he wrote the text. This is evidenced by the following quotation from Vatsyayana's Kama Sutra - "Such passionate actions and amorous gesticulations or movements, which arise on the spur of the moment, and during sexual intercourse, cannot be defined, and are as irregular as dreams. A horse having once attained the fifth degree of motion goes on with blind speed, regardless of pits, ditches, and posts in his way; and in the same manner a loving pair become blind with passion in the heat of congress, and go on with great impetuosity, paying not the least regard to excess. For this reason one who is well acquainted with the science of love (Kama Sutra), and knowing his own strength, as also the tenderness, impetuosity, and strength of the young women, should act accordingly. The various modes of enjoyment are not for all times or for all persons, but they should only be used at the proper time, and in the proper countries and places."

What Was Vatsyayana Trying To Say?

Vatsyayana knew that people were very interested in the study of human sexual behaviors. After all, mankind has not existed for so many years without some first hand knowledge of the subject. However, as an avid scholar of human behavior, he also knew that knowledge of the art of making love was not, in itself, enough to provide for happy relationships. Physical attraction can only reach so far and two people who cannot communicate will not remain together for very long. He also knew that there is a time for everything. There are occasions where certain displays would be unwelcome or even inappropriate.

Throughout the majority of Vatsyayana's text, he tried to show readers of the Kama Sutra how important the emotions and feelings that accompanied congress really were. He advised repeatedly to have an understanding of ones mate and their needs and personality. Without such knowledge and understanding, a relationship would be doomed to failure and unhappiness.

How Does It Apply Today?

Despite advancement and civilization, the human creature is much the same as it was eons ago. We still share the same emotions of our ancestors though our choice of display may differ. What Vatsyayana wrote in the Kama Sutra of his time is still very poignant today. For a relationship to work, more than physical action is required. One must apply themselves to learning their partners quirks and needs. Listen to your partner and act on what you have heard. As Vatsyayana understood so well, Love is made with the heart, not with the body.

The Facts About The Illustrations Of The Kama Sutra

People have spent hours poring over them, trying to mimic intricate poses and styles. Others have had a good chuckle at how well the name of a certain act, such as the tripod or the elephant, matched the aesthetic qualities of the pictorial evidence. Many more just stared in disbelief and said "How did they do that?"

While the illustrations may be thought provoking or titillating, they are not part of the original manuscripts that Vatsyayana penned. The illustrations were added at a later date by translators as a way of making the sometimes difficult wording of the Kama Sutra more readily understood by the average reader and were never intended to be part of the original manuscript, as common myth would imply.

How did the Kama Sutra illustrations get there?

Centuries after Vatsyayana first put the words to the Kama Sutra into the path of history, readers were still interested in his subject matter, perhaps even more so than his contemporaries. Unfortunately for the average reader without a knowledge of the Hindu background from which Vatsyayana had written the masterpiece, some of the language and wording was exceedingly difficult to decipher even though Richard Burton had translated the text into the popular language of the Victorian era of which he lived. People were really interested in the subject matter but, as with many difficult to understand subjects, people shied away from reading long, detailed passages that were hard to comprehend in favor of books which were easier to digest.

This trend continued on for quite some time before someone recognized a need for a change. Proponents of the work and publishers could no longer stand to see the masterpiece shunned because it was too difficult to comprehend so an effort to make the text more readable began. The effort led the way to illustrated copies of the Kama Sutra which we find today.

Where did the Kama Sutra illustrations come from?

The changes of the Kama Sutra had begun. Authors were hired to rewrite the book in the modern vernacular and as publishers decided to add illustrations to the Kama Sutra, they needed to find a source for their illustrations. One such author was Madelyn Carol Dervos who began her rewriting work in 1988 and made repeated trips to India over a period of ten years to collect artwork for her reproduction of Vatsyayana's masterpiece. Traveling all over India and looking at many amazing pieces of art, she sought out paintings that would cause her readers to see themselves in the illustrations and was very successful in this cause. These paintings, as well as others, have since been translated into the illustrations we see in today's illustrated Kama Sutra versions.

Though the so called original Kama Sutra illustrations may not be as original as some would lead us to believe, they do not detract from the work but do tend to enhance the readers understanding of the wording. Illustrated or not, the Kama Sutra by Vatsyanya will remain a master text on the ways of Love.

An Introduction To Kama Sutra Oil

It's a cold, snowy evening. The wind howls outside and whips around the house like a wild beast trying to gain entry to the home. Inside, the house is warm and dry. Soft music is playing in the background. There is a roaring fire in the fireplace, which is providing the only light in the room, with a blanket spread out on the floor before it. You and your partner lay on the blanket sipping a finely chilled glass of champagne and feeding each other chocolate covered strawberries. You have been reading the Kama Sutra and have been utilizing the wisdom of Vatsyayana to restore the fires of passion. In so doing, you have discovered the value of touch and massage as a way of providing intimacy with your partner. Just this afternoon, you stopped at a shop in the next town and bought a selection of massage oils, the Kama Sutra Oils of Love. It is going to be a very enjoyable evening for both you and your partner.

What Is Kama Sutra Oil Of Love?

Kama Sutra Oil of Love is a delectable massage oil that provides for luxurious evenings of gentle relaxation and intimacy. The oils are scented and flavored to increase the pleasure and arousal of both partners by stimulating the sense of taste and smell. These flavorings and scents commonly include chocolate, raspberry, cherry almond, mint, tangerines, strawberries and vanilla creme.

In addition to the olfactory and flavorful pleasures, Kama Sutra Oil of Love also offers tactile pleasures with a warm, tingly sensation and the feel of slippery luxurious oils. These tactile pleasures offer themselves well to an erotic and sensual massage. With the skin being the largest sensory organ of the human body, with literally millions of nerve receptors, massage can be a very relaxing and intimate experience, as well as the physical rewards of reducing stress and toxins in the body.

How Do I Use Kama Sutra Oil?

To make the best use of Kama Sutra oil, it is recommended to warm the product first by soaking the bottle in a bowl of warm water. This preparation can be made while your partner take a hot bath or shower to begin the relaxation process.

When your partner emerges from their bathing routine, make sure the room is warm enough for their comfort and have them lie face down so you can begin by massaging the back. Put a liberal amount of the warm oil in your hands and begin with short, lighter strokes and work up to heavier, long strokes. For the heavier strokes, use your body weight rather than the strength of your arms as this will greatly increase the amount of time you can spend comfortably giving a massage.

Massage involves a few basic motions that can be repeated and switched around in varying patterns for various effects. These key strokes are:

The Glide - This involves long smooth strokes using the entire hand that follows the curves of your partner's body.

The Palm - For this stroke, using the palms of your hands as the pressure points fan out across the body pushing up and then lessening the pressure and returning to the starting point.

Push Pull - This is a simple stroke performed on the sides of the body using both hands, with one hand pushing up as the other comes back in a push-pull motion.

The Lift - This is a kneading, lifting stroke with the fingers lifting your partners skin.

All Thumbs - This stroke is achieved by placing direct pressure on your partners body with the palm of your hand and using only the thumbs pressed against your partners skin and moved in a circular motion.

With these simple motions and a little initiative, Kama Sutra oil can turn a cold, winter night into a very romantic evening.

The Caste System And The Kama Sutra

In every game there are rules to follow and love making in Ancient Hindu cultures had a set of rules all its own. Vatsyayana's Kama Sutra illuminates these special provisions for us so that we might gain a deeper understanding of the principles and ideas that governed the culture of his time. Ancient Indian culture divided people into a caste system with several thousand divisions but four main groupings.. These individual castes had their own ranks and peculiarities.

It is commonly believed that caste's were decided by a persons birth because it was believed that Karma, or what you did in life, affected the cycle of reincarnation and rebirth but it has been show that the caste system was non-hereditary in its original form. While you could interact with people of a different caste, there were special rules of conduct and the practice was generally frowned upon.

To understand how the caste system affected lovers in the ancient Hindu culture of Vatsyayana's time, let us examine the words of the Kama Sutra itself: "When Kama is practiced by men of the four castes according to the rules of the Holy Writ with virgins of their own caste, it then becomes a means of acquiring lawful progeny and good fame, and it is not also opposed to the customs of the world.

On the contrary the practice of Kama with women of the higher castes, and with those previously enjoyed by others, even though they be of the same caste, is prohibited. But the practice of Kama with women of the lower castes, with women excommunicated from their own caste, with public women, and with women twice married, is neither enjoined nor prohibited. The object of practicing Kama with such women is pleasure only."

How Did The Caste System Work?

According to other ancient manuscripts of the time, these castes were divided into four main parts called Varnas. The Varna designations were the Brahmins (teachers, scholars and priests), the Kshatriyas (kings and warriors), the Vaishyas (traders), and Shudras (agriculturists, service providers, and some artisan groups). There was also a fifth classification deemed to be outside the caste system called the Parjanya, Antyaja or Dalits.

These were considered the "Untouchables" as they were considered as being beneath society and this was usually reserved for those with communicable diseases or held occupations that carried communal health risks or severe uncleanness. This grouping would not have even figured into the Kama Sutra because the very presence of such an individual was considered to defile a person of a higher caste. The defiled individual was then required to bathe thoroughly and purge themselves of any impurities.

When applied to the Kama Sutra, the caste system was shown as a way of determining who safe options were for partners. It provided a measure of safety from various communicable diseases between castes as people were less likely to engage in relations with a person who was below them in the caste system.

For those seeking a lifetime partner through marriages, it also provided a way of reducing contention amongst the spouses by ensuring that both families were of the same background and thus had common ground. This also served to keep lower classes from becoming wealthy by profiting from marriages to higher classes as this was most generally avoided.

Chapter 2: Flirting

Flirting and courtship are two very important aspects of any relationship, as without them we would never be able to woo our partner and attract them to us. We all have our own unique style of flirting, some of us being better at it than others, but thankfully the Kama Sutra lays out exactly what we should be doing in order to be the best flirter possible.

Before we dive into the art of courtship and the tricks to up your flirting game, we will break down exactly what flirting and courtship are and how they differ. Flirting is something that is done with a less serious intention in mind than when you court someone. Flirting can be both sexual as well as friendly, and people can engage in it for fun just as much as they can use it to attract a partner. Typically flirting involves using both verbal and non-verbal communication in order to let someone know that you are interested in them. It can involve a wink, touching someone's arm, laughing at their jokes, or any other of ways in which you showcase your interest.

Courting, on the other hand, is more serious in nature and it is dating someone with the intention of marrying them. Some religious beliefs feel that the only acceptable form of dating is courting, while others engage in courting, not for religious reasons but because they are simply at a point in life where they are looking to get married. Courting can, and should, involve flirting, but it is used to win the other person over and entice them to want to marry you. It is never simply used to instigate a fling or sexual encounter, as that would be in direct contradiction to the point of courting.

Now that we have a basic understanding of the two terms, what exactly does the Kama Sutra say when it comes to courting and flirting?

Meeting the Person, You Want to Date

To begin with, the Kama Sutra starts by mentioning that anyone looking to court another should be realistic in their approach. What this means is that any quality that they are seeking in another, they should possess that quality themselves otherwise they have no right to expect it of their partner. For instance, if you want your partner to be extremely good looking, you yourself should also be extremely good looking otherwise you should not put such a demand on someone else. Once you have your expectations in check, then you can begin the processes of searching for your partner.

So, how does one go about seeking out a woman in ancient times when there was no social media and no dating apps? Well, the Kama Sutra suggests the following ways:

• A woman who is ready to be married should be dressed up nicely by her family and placed in a location where she can be seen
• Women seeking a husband should attend events such as sporting matches and marriage ceremonies
• Men should throw parties in which games are played, causing everyone to interact with each other
• Through friendships, two people can then meet and get to know each other
• By asking their parents, a man can have a wife arranged for him

Of course, we can add much more to this list for current times, so if you are at the point in your life where you are looking to meet someone and build towards marriage, or a future in general, you can try the following more common suggestions as well:

• Try going online and joining a dating site - Nowadays there are numerous different sites, all catering to different individuals and desires, so you are likely to find a site that is perfect for you and finding a partner that matches what you are after

• Ask your friends to hook you up with someone - We know the idea of going on a blind date sounds terrifying, but your friends do know you well, so there is always the chance that they might know someone who fits in with what you are looking for

• Participate in a sport or hobby – Take up a new activity that interests you in order to meet new people and also meet someone who shares similar interests with you. Not only will you already have something to talk about, but it gets you out of the house and on a mini-date right from day one

• Take the bus to work – While your morning commute is never fun, why not turn it into an opportunity to meet someone? Public transportation puts you in close proximity with new people that you have never met before.

However, you choose to approach meeting someone, that is only the first step in courtship, as the real work is what comes afterward.

Beginning a Courtship

Once you have found an individual who interests you, who you would like to get closer with and possibly start a relationship, how are you supposed to let them know that you are interested? In modern times, we have many ways of determining if someone is interested in us, and many of these various ways full under the heading of flirting. When we are attracted to someone, either physically or mentally, or both, our bodies automatically respond to them in specific ways. Some of what we do is deliberate, while other actions are completely subconscious and are naturally done simply because we want to be near someone.

Some of the common ways of flirting that you may be more familiar with are:

- Making direct eye contact
- Holding eye contact longer than normal
- Smiling when you look at a person
- Touching them on the arm when you talk
- Winking from across a room
- Complimenting the other person
- Biting of the lip
- Playing with your hair

- Mirroring another person's movements
- Laugh at their silly jokes
- Stand closely
- Stare at their lips
- Keep your arms uncrossed and open
- Tease them playfully
- Drop a witty pick-up line
- Send a flirtatious text message

Sadly, you won't find any of these located within the Kama Sutra as back in ancient India flirting and courting were done much differently. To compare with the above list, let's take a look at different ways in which the Kama Sutra suggests a man flirts with a woman to show her that he is interested and to engage her attention:

- Spend time with her and entertain her with games
- Pick flowers and turn them into a garland
- Cook meals together
- Play with dice or cards
- Playgroup games such as hide and seek
- Do gymnastic exercises together
- Show kindness to her friends

- Partake in services for her maid's daughter to win her over
- Get her gifts that no other girls have
- Give her handmade dolls and wooden figures
- Create temples for her dedicated to different goddesses
- Make her see him as someone who can do everything for her
- Meet her in private
- Tell her exciting stories
- Perform tricks and juggle
- Sing for her and take her to festivals
- Give her flowers and jewelry
- Teach her nurses daughter the 64 forms of pleasure

While many of these sounds a bit strange in today's time, there is a lot we can take away from this list. Mainly, everything described above is meant to make the man stand out from other men that may have an interest in the same woman. This is exactly what modern-day flirting and courting involves as well, as you want to make the other person see what you have to offer and what they will find in you that they cannot find in someone else. Flirting and courting are meant to entice another person, that is their sole purpose, and to let that person know that you would like to be in a relationship with them, or at the very least engage in some sort of romantic endeavor.

Many people get stressed out by the idea of flirting, and so often you will hear individuals remark that they are unable to flirt or are the worst at doing so. This is simply a false idea that they have gotten into them hear, and they are making it into something much more complicated than it needs to be. Flirting does not need to be anything more than smiling at a person you like or going out of your way to do something nice for them. All you are aiming to do is make them feel special and noticed, and to hopefully get them to notice you in return. The best way to go about it if you lack confidence is to simply start off small. You don't need to perform a magic trick or juggle, and instead you can simply compliment their outfit or send them a text asking about their day. The basic act of taking notice goes a very long way as it shows the person you are thinking of them and that you are interested in who they are. Don't overcomplicate things, and let it progress naturally as you feel more comfortable. Once you get outside of your own head, you will find flirting to be one of the most natural acts possible.

A Woman's State of Mind

Within the Kama Sutra, Vatsyayana goes into detail about a woman's state of mind during flirting and courtship and breaks down the different ways she may feel and react, as well as how many should respond to her. Some of the advice is practical and useful even in today's world, but other tips are much more non-consensual and should not ever be utilized. Here are the mindsets that are mentioned along with the details attributed to each one:

A Woman Who Listens but Does Not Show Any Interest

In this scenario, a man should attempt to persuade her by using a middle man instead of just doing it on his own. A good option would be her nurse's daughter or one of her friends.

If a Woman Meets a Man Once and Then the Next Time Is Better Dressed

This indicates that she is very interested, and thus the man will need to do little in order to win her over. If, however, after a long period of time she still does not consent to be with him, then he should be wary but still keep her as a close friend.

When a Woman Avoids A Man Out of Respect

In this scenario, it will be difficult to win her over, but the man can do so by keeping her as a close friend and also employing the assistance of a very crafty middle man.

If a Woman Turns a Man Down Harshly

When this happens, a man should abandon his attempts to win her over and move on to someone else, for she had no interest in anything he has to offer her.

When Meeting Privately She Allows His Touch but Pretends Not to Notice

If this happens then it means she is interested but playing coy, so he should continue on with his advances. It will require extra patience, but he can begin by putting his arm around her while she sleeps and seeing how she reacts. If it is a favorable reaction, then he can continue on by drawing her closer to him and continuing on from there.

If a Woman Does Not Encourage nor Discourage a Man's Advances, but Instead Is Hidden Away in a Place He Cannot Get To

The only option in this situation is to employ the help of someone who is close to her in order to communicate his advances. The best option would be the daughter of her maid. If the woman does not respond to the man through the go-between, then he should reconsider whether or not to continue pursuing her.

When A Woman Proclaims Her Own Interest in The Man

If this happens, then the man can know for sure that she is wanting to be with him, and he can delight in enjoying her fully. In order to realize this situation, however, the man must know the ways in which a woman will show her interest. Ways in which a woman will manifest her love towards a man are:

- She speaks to him without being addressed first
- She meets with him in private
- When she talks her voice trembles
- Her hands and feet will perspire

- Her face will blush with delight
- She will shampoo his body and rub his head
- When washing him she only uses one hand, and instead uses the other hand to caress him
- She stands motionless with both hands pressed against him
- She bends down and places her face on his thighs
- If she places her hand upon him, she keeps it there for a long period of time

The most important thing noted when discussing wooing over a woman, however, is how she responds within the first conversation that a man has with her. The Kama Sutra notes that a man must find a way to be introduced to the woman that he is interested in, and from there he can then carry out a conversation to assess her feelings. By subtle means of flirting, he should try and let the woman know that he has love for her, and if she responds to this in a positive way, then he should continue on with pursuing her over time. If the woman is very open to his expressions of love, and outwardly responds in a favorable manner, then he knows he will be able to gain her over as a wife very easily. Finally, if a woman is open enough to express her love back verbally, then the man will know right then and there that she is his. Vatsyayana believed that this was true for all women, regardless of who they are, where they were from, or how they were raised, and in many ways, this still holds true today.

It may all sound like very obvious information, but when our brains are overtaken by feelings of love, our judgment can become clouded and we may miss some of the most obvious signals that someone else is attracted to us as well. That is why it is important to have them written down in a book like the Kama Sutra, so that even in moments of overwhelming desire we are reminded of the simple truths that come with flirting and courting. Mainly, what we are discussing are various aspects of consent, and how pursuing someone who is not interested in us will not get us very far. While the Kama Sutra often encourages a man to keep trying, it specifies that when a woman harshly turns you down, then it is time to leave her be. You should never force yourself on someone else, and in fact, why would you want to? We all want to be loved and desired, and none of us should settle for someone who dislikes us or isn't as invested as we are in them.

While the Kama Sutra may have some outdated views on flirting and courtship, the basic principles are still applicable even after all of the centuries which have passed since it was written. Take the time to show someone you are interested, go the extra mile, make them laugh, and employ the help of a mutual friend if you are shy are unsure. Whatever you choose to do, make sure you enjoy the process as flirting and courting are almost sport like in their nature. This is when new feelings are blossoming, and a different picture of the future will unfold in your mind. The best thing you can do is to lose yourself in those feelings and to simply see where they take you. Not every person you pursue will work out, but eventually, you will find that one person that appreciates what you have to offer and will offer you just as much in return.

Chapter 3: Intimacy

Intimacy is oftentimes confused with something that is sexual in nature, when in fact intimacy can be displayed in both asexual and non-sexual manner. Friends can be intimate with one another, you can have an intimate relationship with an individual who is not a lover, a certain setting, mood, or location can be intimate, and as most of us are aware, we can have an intimate relationship with our spouse or lover.

But what exactly is intimacy?

Simply put, intimacy is the closeness that you feel with another person and exists within all types of loving relationships. In a non-human sense, intimacy can also be felt in cozy, private settings such as an intimate concert, or intimate dining experience. For the purpose of this chapter, however, we will be focusing on the intimacy felt between two people, particularly lovers, and how to ignite and increase it.

Within intimacy there are four distinct types:

- Physical
- Emotional
- Intellectual
- Experiential

Each one needs to be nurtured within a relationship in order to make it successful, for it is through intimacy that we develop vulnerability, closeness, a feeling of being connected, and a healthier experience. But how exactly do we go about increasing our intimacy? Below we will look at the different ways the Kama Sutra suggests increasing intimacy via touch both by embracing in different ways, as well as through the art of kissing.

Kama Sutra Embraces

Within the Kama Sutra, there are different types of embraces listed that explain in detail how we can hold someone to us. Four of the embraces listed are non-sexual, while the other four are sexual in nature. These unique styles of embracing increase both intimacy and passion and can physically connect two people so that they feel closer to one another both literally and metaphorically speaking. Beyond the eight standard embraces, the Kama Sutra also lists an additional four that forgo the use of the arms and instead focuses on embracing using other parts of the body. In this way, the book goes into great detail on all of the ways in which we can use our bodies to show our love to one another.

Since the Kama Sutra does have a focus on sexual acts, the type of intimacy created through these embraces is one that is more sexual in nature. But, not all of the embraces should be done during a session of passionate lovemaking, and instead, some of the options listed are to be engaged in between individuals who are not yet actively intimate and instead are getting to know each other beforehand. By embracing someone you are letting your guard down and physically letting them enter into your space. You are welcoming them to get to know your body, as well as who you are in the process. Embracing is a very intimate act, and below we will look at the different types and who they should be done by.

The first four embraces listed are external embraces, otherwise known as preparatory embraces. They are to be used between a couple who has come to love one another and are done prior to intercourse although not necessarily as foreplay. Instead, they heighten the intimacy felt between the couple, as well as arouse the man and create an erection.

Sprishtaka – The Touching or Contact Embrace

The first type of embrace listed in the Kama Sutra is the Touching Embrace and it is recommended to be done by individuals who are not yet in a relationship and instead are courting or flirting with one another. This is the least sexual of the embraces and is the common form of hugging that we know today. The Kama Sutra describes it as an action in which a man stands in front of a woman, or to the side of her, and then touches her body with his. He may wrap his arms around her, one arm around her, or simply touch her with as much body contact as possible.

Viddhaka – The Piercing or Bruising Embrace

The second embrace that is designed for couples who are not yet in a sexual relationship but moving towards it, is the Piercing Embrace. This should be done only in a private setting as it is more intimate in nature than the Touching Embrace. This embrace happens when a woman bends over as if she is about to pick something up, and in the process, she pierces a man with her breasts. The man can either be sitting or standing, so long as her breasts hit against him. In response to her action, the man should then grab ahold of her breasts and embrace them.

Uddhrishtaka – The Rubbing or Baring Embrace

This embrace is the first listed that should only be done between individuals who are already open about their intentions with one another and who speak freely about their feelings. This type of embrace occurs either in a public setting or in private, but always when two lovers are walking with each other slowly in the dark. It is here that they should rub their bodies together intimately, creating the Rubbing Embrace.

Piditaka – The Pressing or Squeezing Embrace

Closing out the first four External or Preparatory embraces is the Pressing Embrace. Like with the Rubbing Embrace, this occurs when two lovers are walking together in public or private under the fall of darkness. When they come upon a wall or a pillar, one person should forcibly press the other against it and then the man can press his erection against the woman's body. This is an ideal transition embrace from the External section into the Preliminary Love Play embraces, as it involves the man being erect and can thus lead to sexual intercourse.

Preliminary love play is commonly referred to as foreplay, and Vatsyayana details four distinct embraces that should be used during this period. The first two of the embraces are meant to occur when both lovers are standing up. The final two are meant to be used during the act of lovemaking, which contradicts the fact that they are listed under preliminary embraces as they technically would not occur beforehand. However, as you read the descriptions, you should see that no mention of sex is actually listed, so it would seem that all four can actually be used to create intimacy prior to, as well as during, sex.

Jataveshtitaka – The Twining of a Creeper

The name of this embrace makes it sound creepy, but a creeper is like a vine that winds its way around a tree. So is this embrace, as the woman winds her way around the man and holds onto him closely. For the Twining of a Creeper, a woman should wrap her body around his man in whatever way she sees fit, embracing him while staring at him in a loving manner. She should take his head and bend it down towards her as if she is asking for a kiss, then make the sound of 'sut sut'. While all of this is happening, the couple is engaged in the Twining of a Creeper.

Vrikshadhirudhaka – Climbing a Tree

The second embrace that is listed as one that should occur during preliminary love play is Climbing a Tree. Also done while standing, this embrace features the woman standing with one of her feet placed on top of the foot of her lover, and her second foot pressed onto his thigh. She should then take one arm and wrap it around his back, which her other armrests on his shoulders. The sounds she makes will be that of singing as well as a cooing noise. It is called Climbing a Tree because it as if she wishes to climb up the man in order to kiss him and become intimate.

Tila Tandulaka – The Mixture of Sesamum Seed with Rice

The following two embraces are both listed as ones that should be done at the time of sexual intercourse. As you will notice, both can either be done right before you begin or even utilized during the act to draw you and your lover closer together. In this first embrace, both partners should be laying down in bed in order to begin. Here, the man and woman will entangle themselves within each other by embracing so tightly that each arm encircles the others, while each thigh is wrapped against their partner's. The Kama Sutra goes on to specify that if a man is laying down on his right-hand side, then he should take his left leg and put it in between the woman's thighs. Then, with his left arm, he will wrap it around the woman's right side.

Kshiraniraka – Milk and Water Embrace

The final embrace that is featured under Preliminary Love Play is the Milk and Water Embrace. Mentally, the couple should be in a space where they are both deeply and truly in love and where nothing else matters to either of them. If this is their mindset, then they should embrace as tightly as possible, almost as if their bodies are attempting to merge into one another. This can be done in any position, either with the woman sitting on the man's lap, sitting in front of each other, or laying down in bed.

There are four final embraces that do not involve the use of the arms, and instead are focused on various body parts embracing one another. These embraces can be used during foreplay or during the course of sex as they mostly are comprised of ways of pressing against your lover.

The Embrace of the Thighs

For the Embrace of the Thighs, one partner will take the other's thighs between their own and squeeze them tightly. They can either focus on one of their lover's thighs, or they can place both between their legs.

Jaghana – The Embrace of the Sexual Area

Jaghana refers to the sexual area of the body that exists below the belly button but above the thighs. Both the genital area as well as the anal area are included in this section. For the Embrace of the Sexual Area, the woman will lay on her back with the man laying flat on top of her. Here he will imitate the act of sex by pressing his genitals down against her. He can then engage in any number of sexually motivated actions, such as scratching, biting, slapping, kissing, or playing with the woman's long and flowing hair.

Embrace of the Breasts

The Embrace of the Breasts occurs when a man takes his chest and presses it firmly between the woman's breasts. This can occur while standing or laying down, but simply means that both individuals are tightly embraced chest to chest. There does not need to be any other body parts involved, including the arms, in order to engage in the Embrace of the Breasts.

Embrace of the Forehead

The final embrace that is described within the Kama Sutra is the Embrace of the Forehead. This involves both partners placing their foreheads against one another, while also touching together their mouth and eyes. Intimate and sensual, this is a very passionate embrace that leads perfectly into our next section regarding the different ways in which we kiss.

The Art of Kissing

As we close out this chapter on intimacy, we must take a deep look into the types of kisses that are mentioned within the Kama Sutra. Kissing is seen as something that should occur prior to sex, and Vatsyayana was a firm believer that actions such as kissing, embracing, and scratching are not meant to be used during sexual intercourse. Instead, these are all different forms

172

of foreplay, and as such, should be engaged in with the intention of arousing our partner and preparing them for a sexual union.

Where you can kiss on a person's body is virtually limitless, but in the Kama Sutra, there are strict rules about where is acceptable and where is not. The places listed as acceptable to kiss are:

- The forehead
- The eyes
- The cheeks
- The lips
- Inside the mouth
- The throat
- The chest
- The breasts

Beyond this, the rest of the body is listed as off-limits to kissing, although the author does mention that some regions around the world do also allow for kissing on:

- The thighs
- The arms
- The belly button

It is very important that each person pays close attention to where their partner prefers to be kissed so that they may please them and not cause any distress. Once they are aware of where to kiss, they can then begin practicing the different types of kisses. The varying kisses are broken down into different categories, depending on how they are done and with whom. The first set is designed for young women, as they are gentler and more delicate than some of the other forms described later on.

The Nominal Kiss

The most innocent form of kissing, the Nominal kiss occurs when a woman touches her lips against the lips of her partner but does nothing else besides that.

The Throbbing Kiss

Deepening the Nominal Kiss, the Throbbing Kiss occurs when a woman places her lips gently against the lips of her partner and then moves her bottom lip while keeping her upper one still.

The Touching Kiss

The final kiss described for young women is the Touching Kiss. Here, the woman will take her tongue and touch it against her partner's lip. She should also reach down and grasp his hands within her while her eyes are softly closed.

The next set of kisses is based mostly around head placement and are the typical positions many of us already engage in while kissing. They are:

The Straight Kiss

When face to face, straight on with our partner, this is the kiss that occurs when both people bring their lips together.

The Bent Kiss

For the Bent Kiss, each person should bend their head to the opposite side before bringing their lips together.

The Turned Kiss

Often done by a man to a woman, the Turned Kiss occurs when one partner takes the other by the chin and tilts their head up towards them in order to meet for a kiss.

The Pressed Kiss

The only one that does not involve head placement, the Pressed Kiss is simply when there is more forced used while pressing the lower lip against the lips of the partner.

The Gently Pressed Kiss

This is not a kiss on its own, but a variation on the Pressed Kiss. While the lips are pressed together, the partners should then bring their fingertips and cheeks together and continue to kiss softly so as to refrain from the teeth ever meeting.

An additional eight kisses are listed within the Kama Sutra, each defined as a special type of kiss. These are related to a certain situation more so than being defined by the way in which lovers kiss. The special kisses are:

Kiss of the Upper Lip

The first two are slightly different than the rest, as they still fall under ways to kiss regardless of the situation. The Kiss of the Upper Lip involves the man kissing the woman's upper lip while she kisses his lower lip.

A Clasping Kiss

Sorry to those with a mustache, but this is specified as only being possible by men without one. Here, the woman takes both of her partner's lips and will place them inside of her own. If during a Clasping Kiss one person touches the others' teeth or tongue with their tongue, this is then referred to as Fighting of the Tongue.

Kiss that Kindles Love

When the man is asleep, if a woman looks upon her sleeping lover and wants to show her desire, she will have a Kiss that Kindles Love.

Kiss that Turns Away

This kiss is done when the man is preoccupied with something else, such as work or if he is in the midst of fighting with his lover.

Kiss that Awakens

If one partner works late and the other has already gone to sleep, the Kiss that Awakens is what happens when they come into the bedroom and kiss them softly after returning home.

Kiss Showing the Intention

A unique situation, this kiss occurs when one lover kisses their partner's reflection in either a mirror or some other surface.

Transferred Kiss

This kiss is not done to the person's lover, but instead is done in the presence of them. By kissing a child that sits on their lap, or by kissing a picture or figurine, they are engaging in a Transferred Kiss.

Demonstrative Kiss

The final kiss is done by a man to a woman when out in public. If she is standing, he will kiss her on the finger, but if she is sitting then he is to kiss her on her toe. For women, this kiss occurs when bathing her partner, if she stops to place her head against his leg and kisses his thigh.

Chapter 4: Foreplay

The Kama Sutra goes into great detail about the different forms of actions and sounds that can occur before and during intercourse. Vatsyayana mentions that actions such as embracing, kissing, scratching, and biting are all meant as foreplay and should not necessarily be used during sex. Instead, in the act of sexual intercourse, the partners should only add in striking and sound making in order to showcase their arousal and desire. Since we already covered embracing and kissing in the previous chapter, we will begin this one by looking at the pressing of nails and the art of scratching.

Pressing of the Nails and Scratching

There are eight different types of scratches that are described within the Kama Sutra, each based on a certain way of pressing the nails into the skin.

1.   Sounding – Pressing in the nails so that no mark is made

2.   Half Moon – Leaving a curved mark along the neck and breasts

3.   Circle – Two half-moons created beside each other

4.   Line – A scratch that is made in the shape of a line

5.   Tiger's Nail – A curved scratch made on the breast

6.   Peacock's Foot – A curved mark made by pressing all 5 nails into the breast

7.   The Jump of a Hare – A scratch-made with all 5 nails near the nipple

8.   Leaf of a Blue Lotus – A mark made in the shape of a lotus near the breast

These marks are all designed to be placed in hidden locations across the body, particularly on the breast, so that they are only seen by the two lovers and by no one else. They are there to remind the person of their lover and to excite them whenever they gaze upon each mark.

Biting

Similar to the pressing of nails and scratching, there are eight different kinds of bites that are made by a lover onto the body of their partner. These are also done in private places on the body and are used as a way to remind the partner that they are loved and desired. The eight types of bites are:

1.   Hidden Bite – A bite where no teeth marks are left, only redness in the area

2.   Swollen Bite – When the bite causes the skin to be pressed on both sides

3.   Point – Only two teeth are utilized in order to nip at a small section of skin

4.   Line of Points – Using all of the teeth to bite at small sections of skin

5.   Coral and the Jewel – When you bite someone using both your teeth and lips

6.   Line of Jewels – Any bite that is made using all of the teeth

7.   Broken Cloud – If you have space between your teeth, this type of bit will leave a round mark that is not fully enclosed

8.   Biting of a Boar – Many rows of bites all close to one another

Striking

When it comes to striking a lover, this should only be employed during sex and with the consent of both individuals involved. Not everyone enjoys being slapped or struck, so never engage in this unless you have discussed it beforehand. If, however, both of you are interested in adding in striking during sexual intercourse, the Kama Sutra lays out the rules for doing so.

First, the places that you are allowed to strike your partner are:

• The head
• The shoulders
• The back
• The sides

- In between their breasts
- The Jaghana

You may then strike them in four different ways:

- With the back of your hand
- With the fingers sprawled out
- With an open hand
- With a fist

It is during being struck that a lover will make various sounds, as she may be in pain and so she will cry out. Any blows that one lover delivers, should always be reciprocated by the other. This is never a one-sided activity, and each action should be mirrored in order to highlight the pleasures that are being felt. It is also important that you strike in different ways along different spots on the body. For example, if striking with a fist, this should only be done along the back as it is sturdier and should never be done to the head. Striking should never be done in excess and is not done out of anger but instead out of pure pleasure.

Mouth Congress

We call it by many names, but oral sex is referred to in the Kama Sutra as the Auparishtaka, or Mouth Congress. This act is not discussed in a way that would suggest it is done by a woman to a man, but instead is most often described as something one man does to another. With that said, however, we will discuss the different forms in a way that can be applied to any couple. There are eight steps to proper Mouth Congress, which are:

• Nominal Congress – Holding the lingam in your hand, you then place it between your lips and move your mouth
• Biting the Sides – Using your fingers to cover the top of the lingam, you then kiss and bite along the side of it
• Outside Pressing – Kissing along the head of the lingam
• Inside Pressing – Placing the lingam inside the mouth and squeezing it with the lips before removing it

186

- Kissing – Holding the lingam in the hand, you kiss it completely
- Rubbing – This occurs when you use your tongue and lick all over the lingam
- Sucking a Mango Fruit – Putting only half of the lingam in the mouth and sucking on it
- Swallowing Up – This is when the entire lingam is placed in the mouth and down towards the back of the throat

Types of Sexual Union

Before a couple engages in sexual activity, there are different types of sexual unions that can occur which are influenced by various aspects of each person's body and personality. The two main types that men and women need to pair up within are the type of unions affected by dimensions, and the type of unions that are affected by the force of passion and attraction.

The type of unions affected by dimensions is referring to how a man and woman's genitals physically fit together. For a man, they may have a small, medium, or large lingam which plays a big role in what type of woman they are best suited to have intercourse with. Women also fall into the same three types, depending on whether their yoni is small, medium, or large in size.

Men who have a small lingam are referred to as Hares, while men with medium-sized lingams are Bulls. The men who are very well endowed and have a large lingam are referred to as a Horseman.

Women with small yonis are considered to be Deer, while those who have a medium-sized yoni are Mares. For the women who have a larger and deeper yoni, they are referred to as Elephants.

An equal union is one that occurs between partners whose genitals are the same in size. A Hare should be with a Deer, a Bull with a Mare, and a Horse with an Elephant. Anything outside of these pairings is considered to be an unequal union. For unequal unions in which the man is bigger than the woman, this is called a High Union, but if the man is smaller than the woman then it is a Low Union. The best form of union is one that is equal, but if this is not possible then a higher union is always greater than a lower one.

The force of passion than a man and woman display also impacts the type of union that they can engage in. This refers to each person's sex drive and is categorized as being small, middling, or intense.

Small passion is when the sex drive is low, and for men when semen production is lessened. For those with an average sex drive, they are considered to have a middling passion. If your sex drive is insatiable and full of desire, then you have an intense passion. Similar to unions based upon dimensions, it is ideal that partners have equal passions, for it will better ensure that everyone is satisfied within their sex life.

Acts Done by the Man

During sex, there are certain acts that should be done by the man in order to bring the woman to orgasm. These nine motions are the different ways he can move his lingam in order to create pleasure inside the woman. In addition to the eight acts that he does, there are also three more that are done by the woman in order to enhance sex for both individuals. The eight that men can engage in are:

- Moving Forward – When the man brings the lingam to the yoni directly
- Churning – Holding the lingam in his hand, the man then turns it inside the yoni
- Piercing – The man strikes the upper part of the yoni
- Rubbing – The many rubs the lower part of the yoni
- Pressing – When he presses his lingam against the yoni for a longer time
- Giving a Blow – Taking the lingam completely out of the yoni and then forcefully re-entering
- Blow of a Boar – Rubbing one side of the yoni
- Blow of a Bull – Rubbing both sides of the yoni
- Sporting of a Sparrow – Moving up and down inside the yoni without taking the lingam out

Then, there are the three acts a woman can engage in, which are:

- The Pair of Tongs – Being able to hold the lingam inside the yoni while forcibly pressing down against it for a long duration
- The Top – With practice, it's when a woman can spin around like a wheel while having sex
- The Swing – If the man lifts up his hips, the woman then swings herself and rotates her body

If during sex the man gets too tired, then it is acceptable for a woman to begin to act the part of a man. What this means is that she will get on top of him and continue to have sex while he lays there and rests. This can also be done simply for fun, or to excite the man, and does not need to be reserved only for when he is worn out. Here she should be able to bring herself to climax so that she is fully satisfied.

Types of Congress

During sex, it is important that the man takes note of the woman in order to ensure that she is fully enjoying herself. Some of the ways that you can tell if she is satisfied is if:

- Her body is fully relaxed
- She keeps her eyes closed
- She is not shy or ashamed
- Her body presses in such a way as to bring the lingam and yoni closer together

If she is not enjoying herself, she may show that by:
- Shaking
- Kicking or biting
- Continues after the man has stopped
- Does not let him rise after sex

During the actual act of sex, there are seven different types of congress that the Kama Sutra notes. These are the different situations in which two people may have sex, and can be based on a specific situation, location, or way of having sex. The following are the various kinds of congress:

- Loving Congress – This occurs when the two lovers have been separated for some time, either due to work obligations, travel, or because of a fight. It is done in a way that satisfies both partners equally and can last for as long or as short depending only on what they need to reach climax.

- Congress of Subsequent Love – This is when new lovers come together at the beginning of the relationship

- Congress of Artificial Love – When two people are attached to others, but still have sex with one another

- Congress of Transferred Love – This happens when a man thinks about someone else that he loves during sex

- Congress Like That of Eunuchs – Sex between a man and a woman who is in a lower class than him

- Deceitful Congress – Sex between people of different villages or countries

- Congress of Spontaneous Love – Sex between two people who are married to each other and is done in a way that both enjoy

With all of the above in mind, you are now ready to move on to the actual sex positions that are contained within the Kama Sutra. The next chapter will go in-depth with regards to many different positions and discuss why they are so powerful and pleasurable. Make sure to include everything that has been learned up to this point, including the embraces, kisses, strikes, bites, and scratches in order to fully experience the Kama Sutra.

Chapter 5: Sex Positions

Before diving deeply into each of the sex positions offered up the Kama Sutra, we will first begin looking at the different types of congress based on the depth of the woman's yoni (vagina). As we discussed in previous chapters, both men and women fall into three different categories based on their genital sizes, and those sizes impact what positions are ideal for each person.

For women who are deer, they have a shallower yoni, and thus they will benefit from engaging in positions that open them up to allow for better entry and depth control. Mare's fall in the middle, so the majority of positions will work fine for them. Lastly, Elephant women, who have wide yonis, benefit from engaging in positions that shrink and tighten the vagina so as to provide more stimulation and pleasure for both partners.

The Kama Sutra refers to the different positions as either High Congress or Low Congress or Equal congress. What this depends on is the pairing between the man and the woman and their personal genital sizes.

If a Deer Woman, with a shallow yoni, engages in sex with a Horse Man who is large in size, then that is High Congress. She should then ensure she is in a position that widens her so that she may accept him inside, and the ideal positions for that are the widely opened position, the yawning position, or the position of the wife of Indra.

For an Elephant Woman, with a wide yoni, who engages in sex with a Hare Man who is small in size, she is having Low Congress. This will require her to lay in a way that constricts the vagina making it tighter and shallower. Positions available for Low Congress are the clasping position, the pressing position, the twining position, and the mare's position. It is also advised that the woman uses various medicines to help her achieve orgasm, as the man's size may not be sufficient for her.

Now, Equal Congress happens when both the man's size and woman's size are equal to one another, such as an Elephant with a Horse, a Bull with a Mare, and a Hare with a Deer. In these cases, the couples may engage in sex any way they choose as all positions should lead to equal pleasure among both parties.

With regards to Mare Women, who are middle in size, the same rules apply. If a Mare engages in sex with a man who is too large, she too is engaging in High Congress and should opt for positions that open her up more widely. If she has sex with someone who is smaller in size than her, then that is Low Congress, and like with the Elephant Woman, she should attempt positions that tighten the yoni.

So, now that you have a general idea of which positions may work best for which type of person, it's time to get into the positions laid out in the Kama Sutra. We will look at what each one is, who it is best for, whether or not it is a realistic option, and many other tips and pieces of advice.

The Widely Open Position

The Widely Open Position begins with the woman laying down on her back. She should keep her head low and against the bed, while she raises up her hips so that they are higher than her head. Keeping her knees bent, her feet should not touch the ground, and instead, her knees should touch against the man's upper back. This position is designed to allow for the yoni to widen. Her partner should be kneeling between her legs, raised up so that he can meet her with his lingam. Her buttocks and lower back should rest comfortably upon his knees, while his hands grasp her sides. To bring her up higher, he may grasp on to her buttocks and raise her lower half to meet him. To increase the deepness of penetration, the woman should clasp on to the man's ankles, so that she may pull herself more tightly towards him.

This position is great for women who are with more well-endowed men, as it will open you up and allow for easier entry. But, do not think this position is only pleasurable for High Congress! Regardless of size, the Widely Open Position ensures that not much effort is exerted during sex, so that stamina for both people is increased. This is a very powerful position that can make sex last for as long as you would like it to, and neither person should find themselves getting tired quickly. It is also an intimate position, as the man gazes down upon the woman, and she gazes back up at him. Both people have their hands free if they so choose, so that they may caress each other's bodies. Men should make use of the fact that the woman's breasts are readily available to him, and he should play with them and stimulate them accordingly.

The Yawning Position

The Yawning Position has the woman begin by lying flat on her back. From here, she will need to open up her thighs as wide as possible, and then raise them in the air until her thighs are against the bed, close to the sides of the body. To assist in keeping them open, she should grasp her thighs or ankles and hold them apart. The man will then lay or kneel in between her legs and can begin penetrating her. There are a few variations that are available for this position, depending on how flexible the woman is and how the man prefers to be positioned. In the ideal situation, the woman should grasp her ankles, or her lower calves, in order to ensure her legs truly are spread wide and open. For proper Kama Sutra technique, the man will then be laying between her legs, but this can require a lot of upper body strength, as he will need to position himself on his hands or forearms to keep himself supported and this can get tiring after a while. Instead, you can alter the position by having the man kneel and lean down, which will assist with stamina.

This is another one of the positions that are listed as being ideal for High Congress, as there are few other positions that truly open up the vagina like this one. Here, the woman is as wide as she can possibly go, making deep penetration and larger penises very doable. It is an extremely intimate position, as the woman is completely exposed to her partner, and he can visually take in every part of her intimate area. For some people, this may offer too much exposure, but if you are confident enough to try it out, it can be very sensual and pleasurable. To increase the intimacy and romance, the man may lean down and kiss the woman, as the bodies are lined up perfectly for this. Both partners also face to face in this position, so you can look deeply into their eyes and connect on a more spiritual level. With that said, this position can also be extremely erotic and rough, depending on how you like to have sex. The wideness allows for fast and deep penetration, and the man can really take control here.

The Expanding Position

A slight variation from The Yawning Position also has the woman laying on her back with her legs widely spread apart. The difference that separates the two, however, is that the woman will not use her hands in order to assist her in keeping her legs apart. She may place her hands behind her head in a relaxed pose, or she may use her hands to caress the man's body. Whatever she chooses, she will need to keep her legs open naturally which can get tiring after some time. In order to offset the fatigue this position can cause, the woman can keep one leg sprawled out to the side but resting on the floor, while then raising the other leg up and away from her body. Here she will still be expanded open, but she can switch between which leg is on the ground in order to rest.

Since this position is so closely related to The Yawning Position, it offers all of the same benefits that we mentioned above. From deeper penetration, a wider vagina, and a more visually stimulating position for the man, this is a great position to try out if you are looking to spice things up in the bedroom. But, to truly enjoy both The Yawning Position and The Expanding Position, the woman must be able to leave all of her inhibitions at the door so that she can be confident and let herself go.

The Position of Indrani

Closing out the three recommended positions for High Congress is The Position of Indrani, which is also known as the Position of the Wife of Indra. To get into this pose, the woman will lay on her back and spread her thighs open. She will bend so that her thighs are on the ground on either side of her. Her legs should fold on top of her thighs, with her claves resting on the back of each thigh. This is a very tricky position and requires a high degree of flexibility on the woman's part. If you are unable to master it on your first go, simply bend the thighs back towards the floor as much as possible, and then work towards it over time. Even in the Kama Sutra, it is noted that this is a position that requires much practice, so do not feel discouraged if it does not come naturally to you.

This is the position of the Highest Congress and is the most useful for couples who are experiencing size differences. For larger sized men, this is the best position to assist with penetration, as the woman's vagina is opened up perfectly to allow for insertion. If you are finding the woman is unable to have her legs pushed back enough to make it work, the man should assist her as much as possible, by using his forearms to press down against the back of the woman's thighs. Do note, however, that you should not press down too hard, as you don't want to injure her in the process. Only push as far as she is comfortable, and never force her legs or cause any strain in the process.

The Side Clasping Position

The first of the Low Congress positions, the Side Clasping Position has both the man and woman laying on their side. To begin, the man should lay down on his left side, and the woman will lay on her right side so that she is facing him. Keeping her legs tightly pressed together, and him with his legs tightly together, he should then press himself against the woman's body and enter her from this position. Both the partner's legs should remain in a straight posture for the entire duration, and their bodies should stay tightly pressed against each other. There will be no space for the man to caress the woman's breasts, but he can run his hands along her back and buttocks.

As you may be able to tell immediately, this is a position that makes penetration a bit more difficult. The vagina is closed and hidden between the legs which are tightly pressed together. This is why it is the position of Lowest Congress, as it is designed to be most beneficial for couples where the woman has a larger yoni and the man has a smaller lingam. Surprisingly, however, this position may not actually be as possible for men with smaller penises, as the distance needed to properly penetrate requires more length from the man. We would say that in general, this position is not typically a favorite of most couples, but that doesn't mean it isn't worth trying. If you can accomplish it, it will provide the snuggest fit for the man, leading to increased pleasure for both people. The tightness will ensure that the woman completely feels the man entering her, and the man will feel the woman's vagina hugging his penis for the entire duration of sex.

The Supine Clasping Position

The Supine Clasping Position is actually the main version of the Clasping pair and is a bit easier to engage in than The Side Clasping Position. Here, the woman will lay flat on back, with her legs straight out and pressed together. Think of yourself like a plank of wood, with your body in a perfectly straight alignment. Now, the man will lay on top of the woman, matching her position. His legs should also be straight and pressed together, resting on top of the woman's legs. His body should press down against hers, and he can place his hands on either side of her so that he can prevent her from having to bear all of his weight. The many must then enter the woman from this position, not spreading her legs at all, so that her yoni remains tightly squeezed shut.

If you are looking for depth, this position is not going to be the one for you. Because of the angle of the woman's pelvis, and the tightness of her legs, there is very little room for the man to be able to insert himself. However, if you are looking for a tight, squeezing sensation, then this position always delivers. Like with The Side Clasping Position, this is the position of Lowest Congress, so it is meant for wider women and smaller men. But, as we mentioned above, this may actually not be possible for men who are too small in length, as they will need to make up the distance that is reduced by the woman having her legs closed. Instead, this position is good for men who have more length, but possibly less width. If you fall into this category, you should find that The Supine Clasping Position is quite pleasurable for you.

The Pressing Position

The Pressing Position is less of a position, and more of a move to engage in during The Clasping Position. While the Kama Sutra does list it as its own position, it requires that you are already engaged in sex in order to complete. For this, the couple must already be engaged in either variation of The Clasping Position, although The Supine Clasping Position works best. Once you are engaged actively in sex, the woman will then use her thighs to press down tightly against the man's erection. Living up to its name, she will begin pressing tightly against it, squeezing it so as to add more pressure and tightness for him.

Like the next two positions we will discuss, The Pressing Position is more of a technique that a woman can utilize during sex in order to alter the sensation for both herself and her partner. It may seem unnecessary, given that The Clasping Position already offers up maximum tightness, but it is a tool at your disposal if you are looking to spice things up and play around. This move also gives the woman some control during sex, as she can effectively alter the depth and tightness to suit her desires.

Twining Position

This is another one that is listed in the Kama Sutra that is more of a technique than it is an actual position. The Twining Position can be utilized during almost all of the other sex acts, and simply consists of the woman placing her thigh over her lover's thigh. Two ways in which this can be visualized is by thinking of it in either a standing or laying down position. Beginning with laying down, if the man is on top of the woman, she can take one of her legs out from under him and bring it around the side so that her thigh is then pressed against the outside of his thigh. So long as her thigh is across his, The Twining Position is taking place. For those who enjoy sex standing up, this can easily be achieved in any standing position, regardless of whether or not you are facing each other. If you are standing face to face, the woman should lift one of her legs and place the thigh against the outside of the man's thigh. If you happen to be in a position where the woman has her back to the man, she can lift her leg and stretch it out behind her until she finds his thigh with hers.

What makes this technique so useful is that it is extremely simple and oftentimes something we already do naturally. Many positions automatically place the man and woman so that their thighs touch, so this is just being more aware of that placement. The Twining Position is perfect for enhancing the feeling of closeness, as the deliberate action of touching your bodies together connects you and you can focus on the sensation of your thighs pressed against each other.

Mare's Position

The final technique that is listed under Low Congress in the Kama Sutra is the Mare's Position. Like we saw with The Pressing Position and the Twining Position, this is in fact not a position at all and is instead a way for the woman to increase tightness during sex. What is required here is for the woman to literally trap the man's lingam inside her yoni so that he cannot remove himself. This is going to require the woman to have developed her Kegel muscles so that they are able to be engaged at her will. The Kama Sutra does make a point of saying that this technique is only learned through practice and is performed only by certain women who have been trained in this act.

If you want to be able to engage in The Mare's Position during sex, then you are going to need to train yourself to be able to utilize your Kegel muscles when you like. You will also need to practice strengthening them, as simply squeezing gently will not be enough to trap the man's penis inside you. In order to strengthen these particular muscles, you will need to learn exactly what you are feeling for, and this can be done the next time you go to urinate. While peeing, stop yourself mid-stream by clenching your pelvic muscles, then release and continue urinating. Once you have the hang of this, you can then practice that same motion anywhere and anytime. You should hold the muscles tightly for 3 to 5 seconds at a time, and then release them for 3 to 5 seconds. Repeat these multiple times a day, for at least 10 times per session. For those that want to take their practice a step further, you can actually invest in devices that are designed specifically for this purpose. Yoni eggs are small ball-shaped items that are placed inside the vagina that you can practice squeezing tightly.

The benefits of strengthening your Kegel muscles extend far beyond The Mare's Position, however, and this is actually something all women should practice doing. Strong Kegel muscles can help prevent incontinence as you age, or that can develop from pregnancy and birth. This also strengthens the pelvic floor which can aid in childbirth, as well as preventing the pelvic floor from collapsing post-birth.

Rising Position

The Rising Position is a combination of both a technique as well as a position, as it can involve a wide array of variations to the pose. The basics of The Rising Position involve the woman simply rising her thighs up into the air, and from there the rest is up to you. Since this explanation is extremely vague within the Kama Sutra, we have gone a step farther, but breaking down a few ways in which you can do this pose. By beginning with the woman on her back, she should raise her thighs up into the air and place her ankles on the man's shoulders. He will kneel over her, pressing her thighs back towards her, and then penetrate from here. The other option is for the woman to raise her legs into a V-shape and then simply hold her thighs open with her hands. You may remember a similar position from earlier called The Yawning Position. This is similar in the sense that the woman's legs are wide apart, but whereas The Yawning Position has the thighs pressed back against the ground, The Rising Position keeps the thighs in the air.

For most couples, you may find that you already incorporate The Rising Position in your regular sex routine, as having the woman's legs up in the air in a V formation is quite common. This is a popular position for many reasons, but mostly because it is simple, versatile, and provides great depth of penetration. The more the woman bends her knees in this position, the deeper the man will be able to go, so she can take some control by engaging this technique. Now, the reason we call this more of a technique than an actual position is because The Rising Position encompasses any pose that has the thighs raised in the air. You can approach this from a number of different ways, so go ahead and get creative!

The Pressed Position

The Pressed Position was already mentioned above, when we discussed different ways you can utilize the Rising Position. Like previously described, this position involved the woman lying flat on her back, and then lifting her legs into the air. From here, she should place her legs on her man's shoulders in whatever position she finds most comfortable. Many women will perform this by simply placing their ankles on their partner's shoulders, while others will use their calves or the backs of their knees. Traditionally, this position has the woman resting her feet against the man's chest, a variation that narrows the vagina and makes more a more shallow but tight fit. Regardless of what you choose, as long as your legs or feet touch his shoulders you have successfully gotten into The Pressed Position.

This is such a popular position and many couples find it to be their favorite as it is extremely versatile. If you enjoy intimate sex, this position has you both gazing into other's eyes as he slowly works his way inside you. For those that prefer a much rougher and tumble version of sex, this pose will allow him to grip on to you and really go to work. No matter what your preference, this position can be adapted to suit almost any need and is sure to please both of you immensely.

Half Pressed Position

The Half-Pressed position is a variation of The Pressed Position and involves the woman changing the position of one of her legs in order to create a much loser fit. Unlike its sibling, The Pressed

Position creates more of a narrow vaginal opening which means that the vagina is tighter, and it can be more difficult if the man is very well-endowed. To allow for a bit of an easier time with entry, The Half-Pressed Position has the woman taking one of her legs and removing it from the man's shoulders. Instead, she should move it out to the side, either keeping it up in the air or placing it down on the ground. She can also opt to wrap it around the man's waist so that there is still ample closeness but also more vaginal space.

Most women should find that the easiest way to engage in The Half-Pressed Position is to actually take the outstretched leg and bend it at the knee. Then she is able to place her foot flat down on the bed while keeping her other leg on her man's shoulders. The reason that this modification is ideal is because the woman can now use the flat foot as leverage, pushing her pelvis up to meet the man with every thrust. This can end up allowing for an increased speed, as well as increased depth as your bodies are better aligned and in sync. However, if you want to experience more closeness and deeper penetration rather than increased speed, the woman should then wrap her one leg around the man's waist, bringing him in tightly towards her. This will slow the sex down, but it will also open up in terms of depth to increase penetration.

The Posture of Splitting of a Bamboo

This is one of the first positions we are going to discuss that involves the woman actively participating in order to make it successful. With the Posture of Splitting a Bamboo, the woman will lay on her back with her partner kneeling in front of her. She will place one of her legs on his shoulders, and then stretch the other leg out to the side. The man should insert himself into the woman and begin having sex at this point. Now, here is where the woman will need to begin being more active. The leg that is on his shoulder, and the leg that is stretched out, will switch positions so that the stretched leg is now on his shoulder and the previously placed leg is now stretched out. Getting in rhythm with her man, the woman will continue to alternate her legs back and forth, keeping one on his shoulder and one outstretched at all times. The continuous movement of the legs will alter the angle of the vagina and change the sensation for the man, as well as change which part of the vagina is being hit with every thrust.

We advise starting out slowly with this move until you feel more comfortable and confident. Not only is it difficult to constantly move your legs into different positions, but it can also be hard to time your movements with your man's thrust. The slower you start this, the easier of a time you will have, and you can build up speed as you go. Timing is everything with The Posture of Splitting of a Bamboo, and the more in sync you and your partner are, the better this will feel.

The Fixing of a Nail

Like with The Position of Splitting of a Bamboo, The Fixing of a Nail is another position that involves the woman moving her legs during sex. What makes this one different, however, is the fact that it requires a significant amount of flexibility on the woman's part, and it is unlikely that this position is going to be for everyone. Many thinks of the Kama Sutra as being a book of outrageous sex positions, and this is one of the mentioned poses that will seem crazy to a lot of people. For this position, the woman will again begin by lying on her back, and her man should kneel in front of her. From here, the man will take on of her legs, lift it up, and then begin to move it into a split like position, where the foot is stretching back towards the woman's head. She should then rest her foot against the man's forehead, while keeping the other leg remaining on the ground straight out as normal. If this doesn't sound difficult enough, the position continues on by having the woman continuously switch which leg is flat on the ground and which has the foot placed on the man's forehead.

For positions such as The Fixing of a Nail, which are more complicated and require a lot of flexibility, you can start by only trying the first half and skip out on switching the legs throughout sex. Having your foot on your man's forehead is already going to be a challenge, so if you manage to get that far then give yourself a round of applause. For those that are able to get into and maintain this position, then feel free to try the full pose by swapping the legs throughout. The switching does enhance the position as it alters the angle of the pelvis and gives a new sensation with every move.

Crab Position

For this position, the woman will need to be laying on her back. Once comfortable, she will take her knees and draw them up towards her chest and stomach area. To visualize this position, you will need to imagine what a crab looks like, with its claws close to its body. This is similar to how the woman will look, her legs wide open, vagina exposed, knees by her breasts, and thighs against her stomach. It is both difficult to describe, but it is also difficult to do if you lack much flexibility in the legs. Make sure your partner assists you in this pose by having them place their hands on the backs of your knees. From here they can press down on your knees to help lower them towards the outside of your breasts, thus forcing the thighs up closer to your stomach.

Once you are in the position it is actually surprisingly comfortable. For the woman, her body is drawn up close to itself but there is very little strain placed on any part of her, especially if her partner is assisting her in the placement of her legs. For the man, he will have direct access to her vagina as it will be spread open in front of him. He can now opt to either kneel in front of her or to lay against her and penetrate that way. Whatever he chooses, he should keep his hands around the backs of her knees to ease any difficulty she may have in this pose. The woman will have her hands completely free in this position, making it perfect for her to access her clitoris and stimulate it in the way that she enjoys.

The Packed Position

The way in which a couple utilizes The Packed Position is up to them, but what it must include is the woman having one thigh pressed against her other thigh. The ideal way to do this is to start by having the woman lying flat on her back, and the man kneeling in front of her. Using him for support, she should lift her thighs into the air, and then cross one thigh over the other, causing one leg to be more bent while the other remains straight. Now, the man can place the straight leg over one of his shoulders or choose any other way of placement that feels good to both partners. So long as her thighs are lifted and crossed, you have completed The Packed Position.

This position does require some muscle strength on the part of the woman, as not only is crossing the thighs tricky but keeping them like that can also be a struggle. Make sure you really lean on your partner for this position to ensure that he helps to offset any strain or pressure you may be feeling. The benefit of crossing the thighs, however, is that it will tighten the vaginal opening and create a snugger fit. If you practice this position enough, you will end up with very strong thighs by the end of it, so you can think of it like a workout and a pleasurable experience all wrapped up in one.

The Lotus Like Position

In the Lotus Like Position, the woman will cross her lower calves across one another in order to create a position similar to what is seen during a lotus style sit in yoga. While on her back, she should bring her legs up into the air, either completely or only partially, and then place one calf over top of the other. For a more traditional pose, her legs should be partially lifted, which can be achieved by having her start off with her legs bent but feet planted on the ground. From here, all she needs to do it lift her feet off the ground and then raise her lower legs until she can comfortably cross them. The man will find it easiest to approach this position from a kneeling position, and he should also find that her feet naturally fall against his chest. By keeping the woman's feet on his chest, he can not only support her, but he can use his body weight to push her legs backward making it easier for him to reach her vagina.

For women that are very flexible, or who would like to practice this in a very traditional way, you should cross the legs like you are in a seated position. To get an idea of what this means, start this position by being seated on your buttocks, and then cross your legs over each other as if you were preparing to meditate. Each foot should rest on the opposite thigh, while the calves will firmly press against one another. Once you have this completely understood, simply lay backwards without changing your legs at all. When your man comes to enter you, he will press your crossed

223

legs back against you, and your feet will touch between your breasts and your stomach. As sex progresses, the man can spread the woman's legs apart when he feels necessary, switching up the angle and position freely.

The Turning Position

The Turning Position switches things up significantly, and it is now the man who will need to perform quite the acrobatic feat in order to properly get into this position. For this, the couple should start in a regular missionary style position, with the woman on her back and the man on top of her. Women will need to ensure that their legs are not bent, as the man is going to need a smooth surface to work on. Once sex is well underway, the man is going to lift himself up, remain inside the woman, and then spin himself around so that he is now facing towards her feet. At no point can the man leave the woman's vagina, as he must remain inside at all times. Sound complicated? It is.

How you make this work is going to be very much up to you, as it will significantly depend on the man's penis. His length will play a major role in whether or not this is even possible, as well as the direction that his erection naturally leans. If the man has an erection that is very rigid and points up towards the belly button, The Turning Position is not likely to be possible. Instead, the man needs a more flexible erection that can alter its angle as he turns. If you are not able to turn yourself around during sex without leaving the vagina, don't worry. You can always modify this pose by turning and re-entering if possible.

The Supported Congress

The Supported Congress is the first of the positions we have come to that gets both partners up and off of the ground. Here is a classic standing pose that is fairly simple and is modified depending on your personal preference. To perform The

Supported Congress, have both partners stand face one another. From here, you only need to find something to support you; the Kama Sutra suggests using each other's bodies, a wall, or a pillar. How you engage in sex after this point is up to you. Some options include standing with both feet on the ground and then angling the pelvis so that the man can insert himself into the woman. Another option is to have the woman raise one of her legs up so that entry can be even easier.

One important thing to know with most standing positions is that height differences can really make or break what you are able to do. In many cases, the man is going to be taller than the woman, which means their pelvic regions generally will not line up perfectly. To combat this issue, utilize things around the house to bring the woman up to a taller stance. You can try wearing high heels or standing on the lower part of your staircase if you have one. You can also stand on cushions, a small stepping stool, or anything else that is stable and gives you enough of a boost to have sex more enjoyable.

The Suspended Congress

Like with The Supported Congress, The Suspended Congress is another standing position for couples to engage in. Here, however, the only support the woman will be receiving is from the man who is holding her up. For this position, the man can opt to either stand on his own, or have his back supported by a wall. He will then lift the woman up, cupping her under the buttocks, and have her wrap her arms and legs around him. Now he is able to insert himself and begin thrusting away. It is highly recommended that the man does press his back against a wall, as he will need the extra boost of support in order to maintain this position and not drop the woman. As for the woman, she will have to fully trust the man for support, as the only thing she can do is wrap herself tightly and hold on.

This position is best suited for short bursts of time, as the strength and balance required to maintain it is not very suitable for long durations. Now, the Kama Sutra does add an additional instruction for this position that makes it even more difficult, so it should only be attempted once you are both very comfortable with The Suspended Congress basics. If you want to make it more advanced, however, the woman should uncross her legs from the man's waist, and instead place her feet on the wall which the man is leaning against. Now, she should use her feet to push herself up and down, assisting the man with his thrusts. This is not an easy thing to do, and will require significant leg strength from the woman, but if you want to really impress your partner then give it a go.

The Congress of a Cow

Think of The Congress of a Cow like a raised-up version of Doggy Style. Here, the woman will begin on all fours, but with her hands and feet, both planted firmly on the ground. If you have done yoga before, you will know the Downward Dog position, which is basically what you will be in for this. Once the woman is secure in her stance, the man can then come up from behind her and mount her as if he were a bull mounting a cow. The terminology used may not be the most erotic sounding, but the position is sure to be a favorite.

To alter the tightness of the vagina, the woman can opt between how she spreads her legs, choosing to either keep her feet touching or to spread them wide apart. The leg width will also be determined by a woman's flexibility, as this position can really make you realize how tight your hamstrings are. If you find that it is uncomfortable, or even impossible, to have both your hands and feet on the ground, bend your knees slightly until you find the right position for you. What makes this position so worth trying is that it plays on everything that is great about the traditional Doggy Style position. Not only is it something a bit different, but the pelvis is tilted at a completely different angle allowing for a whole new set of sensations.

The Congress of a Dog

It turns out that everyone's favorite, classic sex position has actually been around since at least ancient Indian times. The Congress of a Dog may sound familiar, and that's because it is. Otherwise known as Doggy Style, this position sees the woman on her hands and knees and the man kneeling behind her. Simple and effective, this is a great position to start, finish, or maintain throughout sex. The Kama Sutra also offers up other variations, such as The Congress of a Cat, which has the woman bringing her chest down lower to the ground while keeping her buttocks up in the air. No matter what variation you opt for, The Congress of a Dog is a versatile position that has been beloved for centuries.

Very few people can say anything bad about this position, other than the fact that it lacks in intimacy. With the woman facing away from the man, there is no eye contact unless she contorts around so that she can see him. There is also a bit of a disconnect between the two partners, as both may feel like they are in their own world during this pose. However, that aside, this position is easy for any level of expertise and requires no special skills or added flexibility in order to perform it. Great for finishing off in, this position allows for slow or fast thrusting and by tilting the hips up or down, can allow for good depth as well.

One thing the Kama Sutra also notes is that if you engage in any of the animal congresses, you should act as if you are those animals. This may not be for everyone, but if you are interested in how the Kama Sutra suggests sex should be, this is a fun tidbit of information to note. This goes for The Congress of a Cow, The Congress of a Cat, The Congress of a Dog, The Congress of a Goat, The Jump of a Tiger, The Mounting of a Horse, The Rubbing of a

Boar, and many more. So, let your inner animal out, and see what creative noises you can come up with.

United Congress

United Congress is far from a particular sex position and is instead a discussion on how many partners are engaging in the act. In this case, the Kama Sutra defines United Congress as sex occurring between a man and two women who both love him equally. This is not simply a threesome between a couple and a stranger but is instead a throwback to ancient times in which a man may have more than one wife. In today's world, multiple wives are not as common, but non-monogamous relationships and polyamory are making a comeback, so those are instances where the United Congress might occur.

How the three individuals have sex is not mentioned, nor does it matter. The only thing that matters here is that it is between three consenting adults who are all genuinely in love with one another.

Congress of a Herd of Cows

Similar to the United Congress, Congress of a Herd of Cows is not a position at all, but instead refers to group sex that involves one man and many women. Unlike with United Congress, love plays no role in this act and it does not matter if they are all united in marriage or if they are simply enjoying each other's bodies only for pleasure. Again, this could be done with one man and his multiple wives, but it also could be a single man enjoying the company of many single women. Whoever it is that is involved, what matters is that there are more than two women and that only one man is engaged in sexual intercourse with them.

Gramaneri

You may be thinking that the Kama Sutra is a bit sexist when it comes to group sex, as the above two situations discuss only one man with multiple women. However, that is not the case as Gramaneri is the act of one woman engaging in sexual intercourse with multiple men. The Kama Sutra states that this can involve a woman who is married to one of the men in the group, or who is simply single and enjoying the company of many men. Unlike with the United Congress and Congress of a Herd of Cows, the

Kama Sutra actually goes into a bit of detail on how exactly this can be achieved. It states that the woman can either engage in sex with one man at a time, pleasuring each of them one after another. Or, she may engage with all of them at once. To enjoy multiple men at the same time, one should hold her while another penetrates her, and a third should enjoy the use of her mouth while a fourth hold her vaginal area. Of course, what you choose to do is completely up to you, but that is one way in which everyone can be engaged at the same time.

This list covers all of the positions that are listed under forms of congress in the Kama Sutra, but it isn't an exhaustive list of positions that are deemed as being related to the Kama Sutra. A quick search on the internet will bring up hundreds of different positions that are related to, or based on, the Kama Sutra and there are tons of different ways you and your partner, or partners, can play.

Many people only think of the Kama Sutra in terms of the crazy and outrageous positions, and those do exist, but many are simply different ways of laying with someone in order to satisfy both people's desires. In a sense, Kama Sutra has become a catch-all term for crazy sex positions, and that really isn't the case when you actually read the original book. Instead, it is a guide on how to properly position yourself based on the length of the lingam and the depth of the yoni so that neither partner leaves the encounter unsatisfied. If you want to get crazy with the positions, by all means, do so. But it is important to understand that erotic Kama Sutra sex is accessible to everyone and does not require special skills or circus training in order to be successful.

101 Positions:

Extracted from
Sex Positions Guide of Lana Fox

Man Trap

This is a variation of the missionary position. The female should lie back on a bed in the missionary position and have the male lay on top. As he begins to thrust, the female can wrap her legs around him and have more control over the speed and pace of sex.

This is great if you just want some simple sex. You can put little twists on the move like arching the back for better stimulation. Wrapping the legs around the male will also get him going a lot faster!

1.

The female should lie on her back in the missionary position – legs open wide and slightly bent.

2.

The male should position himself over the female and face her.

3.

The male can then penetrate the vagina, just as in the ordinary missionary position.

4.

As the male begins thrusting, or when it feels best, the female can wrap her legs around the male and 'trap' him, forcing him closer of allowing some extra room for him to re-position.

5.

Tip: Using a pillow under the female's back can help cause an arch. This will greatly increase pleasure and will make things much more comfortable when wrapping her legs around the male.

Safety Tips

This position can cause a lot of strain on the female's lower back, so make sure support is provided by using a pillow or cushion! Be sure to ask whether your partner is comfortable and not in any pain at any point and don't be ashamed if you need to say something because you are uncomfortable!

The Deckchair

The male should sit on the bed with his legs stretched out and his hands behind him to support his own weight. He should lean back and bend his elbows slightly. The female should then lie back on a pillow facing him and put her feet up on to his shoulders. She can then move her hips forwards and back and begin having sex.

This is an amazing position for very deep penetration for G-spot stimulation.

1.
The male should sit on a bed with his legs stretched out. He can use his hands behind him to support his weight.
2.
He should then carefully lean back and bend his elbows slightly for further support and control.
3.
The female should then position herself by the male's feet, facing him and laying back on a pillow for support.
4.
Once in position, the female can begin moving herself closer towards the male until her feet are up on his shoulders.
5.
Finally, she can move her hips towards his penis for insertion.
6.
In this position, once penetrated, it is best for the female to be in control and thrust her hips back and forth to get the best control and stimulation.

Safety Tips

This position can cause a lot of strain on the female's lower back, so make sure support is provided by using a pillow or cushion! Be sure to ask whether your partner is comfortable and not in any pain at any point and don't be ashamed if you need to say something because you are uncomfortable!

Corridor Cosy

This one can be tricky as you need to be in an enclosed area. The male needs to lean against a wall and needs to shuffle his way towards the floor until his feet are touching an opposing wall. The female should climb down on top of his legs, supporting her own weight. Her legs should be left dangling and she can begin thrusting.

This is a great one for adventurous and exciting sex!

1.

Find an enclosed area with secure structures such as a thin corridor, hallway, or other appropriate settings.

2.

The male should lean against one side of the wall and lower himself carefully by extending his legs outwards to the opposing wall.

3.

IMPORTANT: The male's feet should always remain on the floor and securely in place at the base of the opposing wall.

4.

The female should position herself on top of him and face towards him.

5.

The female can begin lowering herself towards the penis for penetration, using either the walls around her or the male's shoulders for support. The female's legs should be left dangling while she is on top.

6.

Finally, she can begin thrusting back and forth.

7.

Tip: If this position is too taxing on the strength of either the male or the female, consider having the male position himself in a lower position so that the female's legs can reach the floor. She can then use her legs to help support her own weight.

Safety Tips

The male needs to make sure that he can support his partner's weight and that he isn't going to slip and fall to the floor completely. Likewise, the female should support her own weight as best she can to avoid potential injury.

Twister Stalemate

The female should begin by laying on her back with her legs apart. Her partner should kneel down on all fours in between her legs. The female should then lift herself up, wrapping her arms around his chest for support. She should then slowly bring up her legs so her feet are flat on the bed.

This is a great position for deep penetration and stimulating the G-spot!

1.

The female should lie down on her back with her legs apart and slightly bent at the knee.

2.

The male should then position himself in-between her legs, facing her and on all fours i.e. on his hands and feet.

3.

The female should then wrap her arms up around the male's chest for support. This will require some strength from the female.

4.

The female can then bend her legs and begin to raise her hips. Her feet should now be flat on the bed.

5.

Finally, she can guide the penis into her vagina for penetration.

Safety Tips

This position requires some upper body strength from the female. She should make sure to be holding on tightly to her partner as he thrusts.

The Spider

You should start by facing each other. The female should climb on to her partner's lap and allow penetration. Her legs should be bent on either side of him and the male should be doing the same. The female should lay back first, slowly followed by the male, until both heads are on the bed. Now, move slowly and calmly.

This is a great one for slow sex to enhance stimulation before trying to reach climax – a good one if you have a lot of time.

1.

Both the male and female should begin by sitting on a bed and facing towards each other.

2.

The female should then shuffle forward and sit on her partner's lap.

3.

This is the point where penetration should occur. The female must remain on top of her partner's lap.

4.

Once penetrated, the female should slowly lean backwards and bend her back until her head is on the bed. Her arms can then be positioned outwards until comfortable.

5.

The male should repeat this stage, leaning back slowly until his head is on the bed.

6.

The female can then begin thrusting forwards and backwards.

Safety Tips

This position requires penile flexibility, else there is a risk of the male straining his suspensory ligaments!

If you want to find out if the male's penis is flexible enough, have him stand against a wall. Pull his penis gradually down. If the penis is able to point directly down to the ground without causing pain then you should be fine to perform this position, but still be careful.

The female should stay still when the male is initially penetrating her and guide the penis to the vagina. The female should wait while he finds the most comfortable position and angle to thrust without injury.

Speed Bump

The female should lay on her stomach and spread her legs. The male should then enter from behind.

The benefit of this position is that things can heat up and speed up very quickly. It is a great position for getting a little rough or if you're having a quickie!

1.

The female should lay down on her stomach and spread her legs as wide as she can whilst remaining comfortable.

2.

The male should position himself on top of the female with the aim of penetrating from behind, both facing the same way.

3.

Once in the position, the male should use his arms to support his weight while he guides his penis towards her vagina for penetration.

4.

Finally, the male can perform upwards and downwards thrusts.
Safety Tips

This position can cause a lot of strain on the female's lower back,
so make sure support is provided by using a pillow or cushion!
Be sure to ask whether your partner is comfortable and not in
any pain at any point and don't be ashamed if you need to say
something because you are uncomfortable!

Triumph Arch

The male should sit down with his legs stretched out straight.
The female should straddle him with her legs either side and
kneel down over his penis. Once she has been penetrated, she
can lean back until laying down on his legs.
This position can give the female a great orgasm and the male is
able to stimulate her clitoris during sex.

1.

The male should sit down on a bed with his legs stretched out
and straight.
2.

The female should straddle over the male, bending her knees
until over his penis.
3.

Once in position and penetrated, the female can slowly lean back until she is laying down on his legs.

Safety Tips

This position requires penile flexibility, else there is a risk of the male straining his suspensory ligaments!

If you want to find out if the male's penis is flexible enough, have him stand against a wall. Pull his penis gradually down. If the penis is able to point directly down to the ground without causing pain then you should be fine to perform this position, but still be careful.

The female should stay still when the male is initially penetrating her and guide the penis to the vagina. The female should wait while he finds the most comfortable position and angle to thrust without injury.

The Standing Wheelbarrow

For this position, begin in the doggy style position and have the female rest her forearms on some pillows. Her partner should kneel down behind her with one knee bent up to keep himself steady. Once he has penetrated, he should hold her legs and slowly lift her up as he stands.

This position is great if you are just experimenting and just having fun! Otherwise, it is a bit difficult and isn't very well rated for sensation.

1.

The female should begin on her hand and knees, facing away from the male (the doggy style position).

2.

The female can lean her upper body down towards the floor and rest her forearms on a pillow.

3.

The male should kneel down behind her with one knee bent for extra support.

4.

He can then position himself towards her for penetration from behind.

5.

Finally, the male should grab hold of the female's legs, wherever comfortable and secure, and support her weight as he carefully raises to a standing position.

6.

He can then thrust forward and back.

Safety Tips

The male should keep his knees slightly bent when thrusting. If either of you feels uncomfortable during the position, then you should let the other know and try something else! This one isn't for you.

Sultry Saddle

In this position, the male lays down on his back with his legs bent and apart – the standard position when the male is on the bottom. The female should slide herself between his legs, almost at a right angle to his body. For support, one hand should be placed on his chest, the other on his leg.

This position relies on the female rocking back and forth until she can feel him hitting her G-spot. The great thing about this position is that the female is completely in control so is one of the better one if G-spot stimulation is what you need to reach an orgasm.

1.

The male should lie down on a bed on his back, facing upwards. His legs should be bent at the knee and apart.

2.

The female should position herself over the male on her feet or knees, whichever is most comfortable.

3.

She can then lower herself to allow for penetration.

4.

Once penetrated, the female should place one hand on the male's leg, and the other on his chest for support. She can then use these supports to help her thrust and control her stimulation.

Safety Tips

This position can cause a lot of strain on the female's lower back, so make sure support is provided by using a pillow or cushion! Be sure to ask whether your partner is comfortable and not in any pain at any point and don't be ashamed if you need to say something because you are uncomfortable!

The Propeller

The female should lay on her back with her legs straight and together. The male should lie down on top but be facing down towards her feet. Once penetrated, the male should make small motions with his hips instead of thrusting.

This is a very difficult position and takes some practice to master!

1.

The female should lie on her back with her legs straight and together.

2.

The male should position himself on top of her in the 180-missionary position i.e. over the female but be facing her feet. He should, as usual, be using his arms for support to hold his body weight.

3.

The male can then shuffle backwards until he is able to penetrate the female.

4.

Once penetrated, rather than thrusting back and forth, the male should rotate his hips in small circular motions in a 'propeller'-like movement.

Safety Tips

This position requires penile flexibility, else there is a risk of the male straining his suspensory ligaments!

If you want to find out if the male's penis is flexible enough, have him stand against a wall. Pull his penis gradually down. If the penis is able to point directly down to the ground without causing pain then you should be fine to perform this position, but still be careful.

The female should stay still when the male is initially penetrating her and guide the penis to the vagina. The female should wait while he finds the most comfortable position and angle to thrust without injury.

The Lustful Leg

Start by standing close and facing each other. The female should have one leg on the bed and the other on top of the male's shoulder, whilst wrapping her arms around his back and neck for support. Then he should carefully penetrate.

Once in position, this is a great move that feels fantastic! It does, however, require some endurance.

1.

Both the male and female should begin by standing up beside a bed and facing one another.

2.

The female should wrap her arms around the male's neck and shoulders for support.

3.

The female can then raise one leg on to the edge of the bed. The other leg can then be raised up to the male's shoulder.

4.

Once in position, penetration can take place.

Safety Tips

This position requires penile flexibility to avoid the risk of the male straining his suspensory ligaments!

If you want to find out if the male's penis is flexible enough, have him stand against a wall. Pull his penis gradually down. If the penis is able to point directly down to the ground without causing pain then you should be fine to perform this position, but still be careful.

The female should stay still when the male is initially penetrating her and guide the penis to the vagina. The female should wait while he finds the most comfortable position and angle to thrust without injury.

The Waterfall

The male should sit in a sturdy chair. The female can then climb on top with her legs either side of him. She should lean back until her head is on the floor.

The clitoris is very accessible in this position so is great for stimulation during sex. There is also a lot of friction inside the vagina so this is a great all-rounder for reaching orgasm.

1.

The male should find a secure chair and sit on it.

2.

The female can then position herself facing towards the male with her legs either side of him.

3.

The female should then lower herself on to his penis for penetration.

4.

Once inserted, the male should use his hands to support the female behind her back and bottom.

5.

The female should then slowly lean backwards until her head is on the floor.

6.

Whilst performing step 5 above, the male should take care to support the female's weight however necessary, and the female should take care to move slowly to ensure that the male is not experiencing any strain or discomfort.

Safety Tips

This position requires penile flexibility, else there is a risk of the male straining his suspensory ligaments!

If you want to find out if the male's penis is flexible enough, have him stand against a wall. Pull his penis gradually down. If the penis is able to point directly down to the ground without causing pain then you should be fine to perform this position, but still be careful.

The female should stay still when the male is initially penetrating her and guide the penis to the vagina. The female should wait while he finds the most comfortable position and angle to thrust without injury.

A pillow should also be used on the floor to support and give comfort to the female's head during sex.

The Challenge
This is a difficult position (hence the name) and shouldn't be attempted unless you are confident and have tried lots of different positions before – it requires strength and flexibility.

The female should stand on a chair and bend her knees until in the sitting position. She should lean forward with her elbows on her knees. The male should then enter her from behind.

This one is hard to master. If it is too hard for you, you could also have the female simply stand on the ground and lean forward on to a chair as shown in the illustration below.

1.

A sturdy and secure chair should be found for this position. It may be useful for the chair to be against a wall.

2.

The female should mount the chair and stand up, facing towards the back of the chair and away from the male.

3.

She should then carefully bend her knees until in a sitting position.

4.

The female should then place her elbows on her knees, and hold on to the back of the chair with her hands for support.

5.

Finally, once comfortably in position, the male should approach the female from behind for penetration.

Safety Tips

Make sure the chair is very sturdy and you have good footing. The male should support the female throughout and should have a firm hold of the female's waist to keep her steady.

The Supernova

For this position, the female should begin on top of the male on a bed or other comfortable place. The male should have his head near the edge. The female should place her feet either side of him and allow penetration by squatting down on his penis. She can then lean back on to her arms behind her.

The female should rock back and forth until she can feel herself reaching climax. When reaching climax, she should lean forward on to her knees and shift the male's upper body off the edge of the bed until she reaches orgasm.

This position is all about timing, but if done right can be really fun and give a great orgasm.

1. The male should begin by lying down, facing upwards and with his knees slightly bent and apart. His head should be near the edge of the bed.

2. The female should place her feet either side of the male's waist and squat down in a straddle position for penetration to take place.

3. The female should then place her hands and arms behind her on the bed and lean backwards. Her arms should be locked and providing most of the support.

4. She can then begin thrusting back and forth.

5. When approaching orgasm, the female should launch her upper body forward and on to her knees. This should slightly shuffle the male's head and upper body off of the bed.

6. Tip: Ensure that the timing is right with the once – it might take some practice. But, once done correctly, this can lead to a fantastic orgasm.

Pirate's Bounty

This position is great when you and your partner want to go a bit more out there to reach orgasm. It allows for deep penetration and total clitoral stimulation so is amazingly efficient at getting you to an orgasm.

To get in this position, the female should lay down on her back and the male should kneel in front of her. She should place one leg on her partner's shoulder and the other around his thigh. A pillow can also be used under the female's back to provide support.

1.

The female should lie on her back facing upwards towards the ceiling with her legs apart.

2.

The male should kneel in front of her, facing towards her.

3.

The female should place one leg up on the male's shoulder (whichever is most comfortable) and the other leg should remain beside his thigh.

4.

A pillow should be placed under the female's back to provide support and place her in an arch to increase stimulation.

5.

The male should then penetrate the female.

6.

Whilst having sex, either the male of the female can easily stimulate the clitoris for further stimulation. This is best done when the female is approaching orgasm.

Advanced Doggy Style

This is a simple variation of the traditional doggy style, but with a much better chance of achieving an orgasm.

To do this, assume the normal doggy style position and guide the female's head until it is against the bed. Her back should be bent slightly with her bum in the air. Now, place a pillow or blanket under her stomach to rest on. Make sure the female is relaxed. Thrust downwards at a hard and steady pace for several minutes until she reaches orgasm.

1.
The normal doggy style position should be assumed by both the male and the female - the female should be on her hands and knees, facing away from the male.

2.
The female should allow for a slight inwards arch in her back i.e. she should raise her bottom and chest whilst allowing her stomach to arch inwards towards the bed.

3.
A pillow or large blanket should be placed under the female's stomach for her to rest on and she can then lower her upper body closer to the surface of the bed.

4.

Finally, the male can penetrate from behind.

5.

The male should continuous thrust in a firm downwards motion at a steady pace of several minutes. His motion should become faster and harder as the female approaches orgasm.

G-Spot Missionary

Assume the normal missionary position. Then place the female's legs on to the male's shoulders. A pillow should be placed under her lower back for support and comfort. Slightly push forward until the female's bum lifts off the surface of the bed. Begin thrusting hard at a consistent pace. You can bring yourself closer to her to be more intimate or further away to thrust harder.

1.

The female should lie down on her back, facing upwards with her knees slightly bent and legs apart. A pillow should be placed beneath the female's back to create an arch and provide support.

2.

The male should position himself on top of the female, facing her and using his arms to support his body weight.

3.

The male should penetrate the female just as he would in the ordinary missionary position.

4.
Once inserted, the male should slightly push forward (before thrusting) in order to raise the female's bottom slightly off the surface of the bed. The female's bottom should remain elevated from the surface of the bed throughout.

5.
Finally, the male can begin thrusting at a constant and firm pace.

6.
Throughout this position, the male can slow down his thrust and bring himself closer to the female for intimacy, and lift away from the female for harder and faster thrusts as she approaches orgasm.

Flatiron
The female should lie face down with her hips slightly elevated. A pillow should be used for support under her stomach. She should spread her legs out and straight. The male should mount her from behind with his legs on the outside of hers and penetrate. This position allows for easy access for anal sex or

vaginal intercourse, but limits access to the clitoris so keep that in mind if you need clitoral stimulation.

1.

The female should lie face down on a bed with her hips slightly elevated. Her legs should be comfortably apart.

2.

A pillow should be placed under the female's stomach for support.

3.

The female should now spread her legs further apart and keep them straight.

4.

The male can then position himself on top of the female using his arms for support.

5.

Once in position, the male can penetrate the female virginally or anally and begin thrusting. His legs should on the outside of the females, but they can remain on the inside if the male finds this uncomfortable.

6.

The male is now in control and can build up to a hard thrust.

The Sunday Afternoon

This is a much easier position to try when you want to reach an orgasm. It's a great choice for easy access to the clitoris if you need clitoral stimulation to reach climax. It is a variation of an X position, like The Scissors.

The male begins laying on his side and the female on her back. She puts one leg over his outer-side hip and the other wrapped around his lower leg to pull him close in. The male gently penetrates and begins thrusting upwards.

1.

The male should lay down on his side beside the female. The female should begin by lying on her back.

2.

The female should then place her outside leg over the outer-hip of the male. The other leg should then wrap around the male's lower leg. At the end of this movement, the female should have transitioned from being on her back to being on her side, facing the male.

3.

The female can then use her legs to bring the male in close and allow for penetration.

4.
The male can then gently begin thrusting towards the female in an upwards motion.

Mastery
This is a version of the cowgirl position and doesn't ask for too much physical effort from either partner, but give the male easy access to the clitoris and the breasts for stimulation during intercourse.

The male and female should face each other in the cowgirl position, with the female seated on his lap. Her legs should be kneeling outside his. The position allows for couples to get close during sex and lean back for new sensations.

1.
The male and female should assume the cowgirl position. This is achieved by the male lying on his back with his knees slightly bent and his legs slightly apart. The female can then straddle on top of the male's hips.

2.

The female should transition so that she is in the same position, but resting on her knees rather than her feet.

3.

The female should take control of allowing penetration by guiding the male's penis inside of her.

4.

This position allows for a lot of variation depending on how the female is feeling during intercourse. She can lean forwards to come close to the male for intimacy, sit upwards for firmer thrusts or lean backwards using her arms for support when approaching orgasm for G-Spot stimulation.

5.

When leaning back, the male also has very easy access to provide clitoral stimulation.

Scissors

This is an X position and can be a challenge for those not willing to commit to it. The female should lay down on her back and her partner should enter her from the sides – her clitoris should be up against his top leg.

1.

The female should lie down on her back, facing the ceiling.

2.

The female should ensure that her legs are open wide to allow access by the male.

3.

The male should begin in a sideways position away from the female with his feet in the same place as the female's.

4.

The male can then begin moving towards the female between her legs.

5.

As the male approaches, the female should raise her back and bottom to allow the male's lower leg to be positioned underneath.

6.

As the male shuffles closer to the vagina, the female should help by positioning herself closer to allow for penetration – the female's clitoris should be up against the male's outer leg's thigh.

7.

Penetration can now take place.

8.

Once both the male and female are comfortable, both can begin gently thrusting towards each other.

The Dirty Dangle

Begin by having the female lay down on her back at the foot end of the bed. Have the male mount on top in the missionary position. The female should start moving back little by little until her head, shoulders and arms flay off the back of the bed towards the floor. The excitement of this position can be a new experience for lots of people and encourage orgasm.

1.

The female should lie down on her back at the foot end of a bed.

2.

The male should mount on top of the female in the missionary position, using his arms to support his weight.

3.

Once in position, the female should start shuffling slowly backwards until her head, shoulders and arms flay off the back of the bed towards the floor.

4.

Both the male and female should support each other during the above movement to ensure both are secure.

5.
The male can then penetrate and begin thrusting.

6.
The increased blood flow to the female's head aims to provide a greater and more fulfilling orgasm. This can be done before or during intercourse.

Lazy Male
With this move, there is less thrusting involved and move up and down motions. There is lots of eye contact which can bring you closer to your partner and increase your chance of reaching an orgasm together.

For this position, the male should prop his body up with some pillows against a wall or the headboard of the bed. Here you can control the rhythm of sex. Have the female sit in the cowgirl position with her legs wrapped around his body and stay up and close.

1.
The male should sit up against a wall or the headboard of a bed, using pillows for support.

2.

The female should position herself above the male's hips and squat down to a straddle position.

3.

The female can then transition into a kneeling straddle position and allow for penetration.

4.

The female can then control the rhythm of intercourse as she begins thrusting up and down.

Face Off

Have the male sit down on the edge of the bed or sofa. The female should sit down on his lap, facing him. From here there should be a lot of friction on the clitoris which is great for reaching orgasm if you need direct clitoral stimulation to reach an orgasm.

1.

The male should find a sturdy bed or sofa and sit towards the edge.

2.

The female should position herself over him with her legs either side and lower herself down on to his lap facing him.

3.
As the female lowers herself, she should reach a kneeling position with her legs either side of the male.

4.
The female can then allow penetration by guiding the penis towards her vagina.

5.
During this position, the female should thrust forwards to increase the friction on her clitoris and achieve the maximum stimulation possible.

The OM
For this position, have the male sit down with his legs crossed while the female sits on his lap, facing him. Next, the female should wrap her legs around him and his legs should be wrapped around the back of her, still crossed. Pull each other close together and rock back and forth. You should look each other in the eyes as you climax.

1.

The male should sit down, either on a bed or the floor, with his legs crossed.

2.

The female should position herself over the male and be facing towards him.

3.

The female should wrap her legs around the back of the male's bottom and cross them over behind him.

4.

Penetration can now take place.

5.

Once penetration has been achieved, both the male and female can pull each other close and rock and forth.
This is an intimate position and encourages both partners to remain close. The aim is to achieve good eye contact as the female approaches orgasm.

The Sea Shell

Have the female lay down on her back with her legs raised up and out. The male should lie on his stomach on top and be facing her as he penetrates, just like the missionary. The female's legs should be far apart to allow deeper penetration for

G-Spot stimulation. It will also allow for some clitoral stimulation as he is on top.

1.

The female should lie down on her back with her legs raised up and apart. She may use her arms flat on the bed to support her or hold on to both legs until the male is in position.

2.

The male should lie down on his stomach and face her, much like the missionary position.

3.

Using his arms to support his weight, the male should guide his penis towards the vagina for penetration.

4.

The female should keep her legs wide apart during intercourse.

5.

Once the male is in position, he can push forward to help keep the female's legs up in the air. She can then use her arms for support by placing them flat on the bed beside her.

Squat

This is a simple and commonly used position. The male should lay on his back on top of a bed. The female should straddle on top and lower herself slowly, guiding the penis into her vagina.

The female is again in control in this position and should raise herself up and down, using the bed or the male's chest to support herself.

There is a reason that this is one of the most used positions – it's great for sensation! And gives the female a good workout. The male also has quite easy access to the clitoris to help stimulation when reaching orgasm.

1.

The male should lie on his back at the top end of a bed, legs only slightly apart and straight.

2.

The female should position herself over his waist and lower herself in a squatting position.

3.

Once in position, she should guide the penis inside of her.

4.

Once inserted, the female can raise herself up and down at her decided pace.

5.
The female should be squatting with her feet on the bed in this position i.e. not on her knees.

One Up
This is an oral sex position. The female should lay on a bed with her rear close to the edge. She should raise one of her legs and hold it in position by wrapping it around her thigh. The male should kneel down between her legs and get down on her!

1.
The female should lie down on a bed with her bottom very close to the edge.

2.
The female should then raise one of her legs up into the air and wrap her foot around her other thigh.

3.
The male can then kneel down on the floor facing towards her. The male should grab hold of the female's body and engage in oral sex.

4.

During this position, the female is able to shift her bodyweight to dictate where the male stimulates her.

This is great foreplay before sex.

Face to Face

In this position, you should sit opposite your partner and the female should slide herself on to the male's lap and sit on top of him. She should wrap her legs around his body until they are touching behind him. The male should then do the same and cradle her bum. Rock back and forth together and get close!

1.

Both the male and female should sit opposite each other and face towards one another.

2.

The male should cross his legs and allow the female to shift on top and sit on his lap.

3.

The female should wrap her legs around the male until her feet are touching behind him. She can then allow for penetration.

4.

Once inserted, the male should also wrap his legs around the female and cradle her bum with his hands.

5.

Both the male and female should now rock back and forth for intimate and close intercourse.

This is a great one for getting intimate – it is a slow pace position and is great for stimulation building up to an orgasm. There is also a lot of clitoral stimulation during this one.

The Stand-Up

The female should turn and face a wall several feet away with her bum slightly suck out. The wall should be used as support. The male should then gently insert his penis – he can bend his knees to lower himself if there is difficulty finding access!

1.

The female should turn and face a wall several feet away from her.

2.

The female should lean forwards and rest her forearms against the wall for support. Her bottom should be slightly tucked out.

3.

The female may slightly bend her knees for additional comfort if necessary.

4.

The male should approach the female from behind. He should grab hold of her waist and slowly penetrate. The male may also find that he needs to bend his knees slightly before penetrating if there is difficulty getting access from behind.

5.

The male can then thrust back and forth. He may hold on to the waist of the female. He may also hold on to her shoulders with his arms straight. If so, the female should slightly arch her back inwards.

The great thing about this is that the female can thrust backwards as the male is thrusting forwards so you can both control the speed of things!

Hobby Horse

This position requires a chair. Make sure it is reliable and strong.

The male should lay back down on the chair, keeping his body parallel to the ground. The female can then saddle up facing away from him and with her feet on his knees.

1.

The male should lie with is back down across the body of a chair. He may use his arms to support him by placing his hand firmly on the floor. His feet should be firmly on the floor.

2.

The female should then position herself with her legs either side of the male's waist (facing away from him) and squat to allow penetration.

3.

The female should then lean back and rest her hands on either the male's chest area or on the edges of the chair itself.

4.

Finally, the female should bend her knees and lift her legs so that her feet and resting on the male's knees.

5.

The female can then thrust back and forth to engage in intercourse.

6.

Once the female is in position, instead of keeping his hands on the floor, the male may grasp hold of the female's waist/ breasts for support and stimulation.

This move requires a lot of core strength from the male to hold the position but is a fun one where the female is in control.

The Elevator – Practice Makes Perfect

This is an oral sex position so is great for foreplay.

The male should be standing and the female kneeling in front. This is a basic oral sex position. Be sure to mix up the speed during oral sex to make the experience better for the male.

1.
The male should start by getting into a standing position.
2.
The female should then kneel in front of him, facing him.
3.
The female can then engage in oral sex.
4.
The is a very versatile position and the female is free to alter the speed and sensations she provides the male during oral sex. She may also use her hands whilst doing so.
5.
Alternatively, the male may thrust towards the mouth of the female while she holds her head steady. She may also benefit from the male using his hands to help hold her head in place.

The more you practice, the better you get!

Carpet Burn

In this position, the male should be kneeling down on a carpet, bringing one knee in front of him. The female should then kneel down in front of him and move to allow him to penetrate her. She should use his body for support and both can begin to thrust.

1.
The male should kneel down on a carpet with one knee bent out in front of him.
2.
The female should kneel down in front of the male, facing him. The female should also have one knee bent out in front of her but this must be the opposite knee to the male.
3.
The female should then shuffle towards the male and slot herself between his knees; her bent knee outside of his knee on the floor, and her knee on the floor inside of his bent knee.
4.
Once in position, she may allow penetration and both can thrust towards one another.

BEWARE OF CARPET BURN. The name says it all although that's where the excitement comes from!

The Lotus Blossom

The male should go first, sitting with crossed legs. The female straddles on top and wraps her legs around him tightly. She can begin moving once he has penetrated, and he can help by raising her up and down.

1.
The male should begin by sitting with his legs crossed.
2.
The female should then sit on his lap and allow penetration while facing towards him.
3.
The female should then very tightly wrap her legs around the male.
4.
Once in position, the male should place his hands underneath the female's bottom and help raise her firmly up and down, pulling her towards him on the way back down.

In this position, the male has easy access to the female's upper body so is great for kissing and being intimate. Just make sure you are both comfortable before you begin!

Bridge

The male should lay across two sturdy objects with his body hanging between them. The female should sit on top of him from the side. She should then slowly bring one of her legs up and over so that she is now facing outwards to the side of her partner.

1.
The male should lay across two study objects (such as two fixed countertops) and allow his body to hang between them. The male should face upwards towards the ceiling and may require pillows/ blankets for comfort on his shoulders and legs.

2.
The female should mount on top of the male with her legs either side of his waist.

3.
The female can then allow penetration.

4.
The female should slowly raise one of her legs, using the male's body for support, and bring her leg over to the side so that she is now facing sideways from the male. It may help to imagine sitting on a park bench looking outwards.

5.
Finally, once in position, the female can begin rocking back and forth gently or rotating her hips in a circular motion.

Golden Arch

In this position, have the male sit down with his legs straight, leaning back supporting his weight with his arms out behind him. The female should then sit on top of him and slide herself on to the penis, carefully. She should then bend her knees with her feet situated behind him and begin rocking back and forth.

1.

The male should sit down with his legs out straight.

2.

The male should lean backwards with his arms out straight behind him for support.

3.

The female should then position herself above the male's waist and squat down for penetration. Once penetrated, she should lean back with her arms straight out behind her for support.

4.

Finally, the female should position her legs behind the male by bending her knees and placing her feet towards where his hands are situated on the bed.

5.

Once in position, the female can begin rocking back and forth.

This is a great position as you can both see each other's bodies and have complete control over the speed and depth of penetration.

Spin Cycle

This is a fun one! The male should sit on top of a washing machine with the setting that makes the most vibration. The female should saddle up on top of him, facing away and help him access the vagina.

1.

First, the male should sit on top of a washing machine. The washing machine should have a load on already when trying this position!

2.

The female should position herself by standing in front of the male and facing away from him.

3.

The female can then begin moving backwards until she is able to saddle up on top of the male.

4.

The female should help guide the penis in for penetration.

5.

The male may use one arm behind him on the washing machine for support, and the other can be used to stimulate the clitoris. Alternatively, both arms can be placed behind for support.

This position gives deep penetration with the added benefit of vibrations from the washing machine! This will quickly bring you both to orgasm. If nothing else, the excitement of having sex outside of the bedroom is a great benefit in itself!

Female on Top

The male should lay down on his back with his legs out in front of him. The female should then climb on top and let him penetrate her. She can then lean back to hold on to his ankles or come forward to get close and intimate.

1.

The male should lie down on his back with his legs out in front of him.

2.

The female should position herself above the male's waist and squat down for penetration. At this point, the female should transition from the squatting position to kneeling with one leg either side of the male. She should be facing towards him.

3.

Once in position, the female is free to come close, sit up or lean back and place her hands on the male's feet for support and control. If she does so, she will easily be able to stimulate her clitoris herself.

This is a good one for the female as she is in control of everything. He can also have a great view of her body during sex.

The Manhandle

For this position, the female should stand in front of the male and face away in a position that provides easy access for penetration. The male should then enter her (this is usually easiest when the female is bent over). She should then slowly straighten up, making sure that the penis remains inside her. When you are both ready and comfortable, start thrusting.

1.

The female must start by standing in front of the male but facing away from him.

2.

The female should then bend over slightly with her bottom outwards.

3.

The male can then approach from behind for penetration, holding on to the female's waist for support.

4.

Once inserted, the female should begin slowly standing up straighter.

5.

The male can then begin thrusting.

6.

The male is able to have easy access to kiss the female's neck and stimulate both the breasts and the clitoris in this position. The female is also able to reach behind and grab the male's head to bring it forward for kissing and getting intimate.

The benefit of this position is that it can be done anytime, anywhere! With or without furniture. Inside or out. It is great on if you are able to reach orgasm through different types of stimulation.

Crossed Keys

The female should lay down with her bum near the edge of the bed. She should cross her legs and raise them up into the air. The male should then stand in front and penetrate her. He can then play with her legs during sex, crossing and uncrossing them to change things up a bit.

1.

The female should sit on the edge of a bed with her feet on the floor.

2.

The female should then lean right back until she is laid on the bed.

3.

Now, the female can raise her legs and cross them. Her legs should be lifted right up into the air causing a slight elevation of her bottom.

4.

The male can now approach from her front for penetration. He should hold the female's legs whilst doing so.

5.

Finally, whilst having intercourse, the male should play around with her legs, crossing and uncrossing them when he pleases for different sensations.

This position can offer alterations quickly during sex to change the depth of penetration and offer different sensation. This one feels great.

Melody Maker

You will need a chair or something similar to start this position. To begin with, the female should sit on the chair and lean back to point her head downwards. The male should then kneel between her legs and penetrate the vagina. He should hold her hands to offer support if she needs it.

1.

The female should sit down on a chair.

2.

She should then lean right back until her head is pointing downwards (this might take some core strength!).

3.

The male should then kneel down and approach her for penetration.

4.

Once inserted, it is best to hold on to each other's hand for support and intimacy. This will also maintain stability when things get going.

The idea behind this position is that it increases the blood rush so the female can have an incredible orgasm!

The Peg

The male should begin by laying on his side. His legs should be stretched. The female can then curl on to her side in the opposite direction so that her head is top and tail with his. She should bring her knees up to her chest and put her legs around outside his. He can then penetrate her.

1.

The male should lay down on his side on a bed with his legs stretched out straight.

2.

She should also lay down on her side in the same position. However, the female's head should be where the male's feet are and she should be facing him.

3.

Finally, the female should curl up by bringing her knees up to her chest.

4.

From this position, the male should penetrate and slowly begin thrusting.

This does seem confusing, but once you try it, it will make a lot more sense and you will soon be able to get in position in no time!

Galloping Horse

The male should sit on a chair and stretch out his legs. The female should sit on top of him and slide down on to his penis. Her legs should be stretched out behind him. He should hold on to her arms to allow her to lean back. The female can then bring herself forward and back during sex.

1.

The male should sit on a sturdy chair with his legs stretched out straight.

2.

The female should position herself over the male facing him. She can then lower herself on to his penis for insertion.

3.

Once inserted, the male should hold on to the female's hands in a firm grip.

4.

Finally, the female should extend her legs out behind the male and the chair. She can then lean right back and begin thrusting back and forth.

5.

Ensure that both partners are always holding on to one another's hands as the female is leaning back! She can also use this grip to launch herself forward as she reaches orgasm and wrap her arms around his shoulders for intimacy and support.

This position can offer the male a great view while also giving the female deep penetration. This one is a win/ win position.

Edge of Heaven

The male should begin by sitting on the edge of a bed or on a chair. His feet should be down on the floor. The female would then climb on top of his lap with her legs either side of him. You can hold each other's hands for support and stop you from falling backwards.

1.

The male should begin by sitting on the edge of a bed or on a chair.

2.

The male's feet should be down on the floor.

3.

The female can now, whilst facing him, mount herself on the male's lap with her legs flaying out either side of him.

4.

Both partners should hold each other's hands for support so that neither fall backwards.

5.

Alternatively, the female can hold on to the male's shoulders while he places his hands out behind him to support his weight.

In this position, both partners can move as slowly or as quickly as you like. It is a great one for deep penetration and G-spot stimulation. It is also a good one for staying in sync with your partner as you are both supporting each other.

Reverse Spoons

Lay in bed with your partner and both face the same way. He can then spoon her from behind and can begin thrusting. This is a simple position that is good for intimate sex.

1.

The female should begin by laying on her side slightly curled up so that she does not lose balance.

2.

The male should assume the same position from behind. Both the male and female should be facing the same way.

3.

Once in position, the male can penetrate the female from behind. It may be helpful if the female raises her outer leg while he penetrates.

4.

Once inserted, the male can begin thrusting. The female can also thrust back towards the male.

Good Spread

The male should lay down on his back. The female should then sit on top of him and slide down on to his penis, slowly starting to spread her legs as wide as she can.

The female is in control in this position – the wider her legs are the deeper the penetration will be.

1.

The male should lie down on his back with his legs slightly apart and bent.

2.

The female should position herself over the male's waist facing him. She can then squat down to allow for penetration.

3.

The female should lean back slightly using her arms for support either on the bed or on the male's legs.

4.

Finally, the female should open her legs as wide as possible for deeper penetration and a great view for the male.

The Bullet

The female should lay face up on a bed and have her legs going straight up at a right angle to her body. The partner should kneel behind and start to thrust, using the upright legs as leverage. He can push the legs close together to get a better sensation inside of you, or further apart for deeper penetration.

1.

The female should start by lying flat down on a bed facing the ceiling.

2.

She should raise her legs up to a right angle from her body.

3.

The male should then position himself in front of the female on his knees.

4.

The male can then shuffle forward for penetration. It may be easier if the female slightly lifts her bottom up while this happens.

5.

Finally, the male can begin thrusting.

6.

Whilst having intercourse, the male can use the female's upwards legs as leverage to get harder thrusts. He can also close her legs together whilst they are in the air so that he gets a better sensation himself.

A general rule of thumb – the wider the legs, the deeper the penetration; the tighter the legs, the better the sensation for the male!

Kneeling Dog

The female should get down on her hands and knees and lean forward on to her arms. The male can get behind in the doggy position and the female can sit back on to his lap.

1.

The female should begin by getting down on her hands and knees on a bed or on the floor.

2.

She should then lower her arms so that she is bent down closer to the floor. Her bottom should remain in the same position up in the air.

3.

The female should slightly arch her back inwards ensuring that her bottom remains up.

4.

The male can now kneel down behind her and approach her for penetration.

5.

Once inserted, the female can lift her body back up slowly until she is kneeling on his lap and begin thrusting back and forth. The male has very good access for breast and clitoral stimulation in this position.

Alternatively, the female can remain with her body close to the floor and thrust in an upwards and downwards motion. It's best to mix up to two different variations during sex!

This is a great one for the male and will really get him going! It also allows for great penetration and friction with the vagina so is one of the best! You might want to write this one down...

Back Breaker

The female should lay on a bed with her legs off the edge as well as her bum. The male should kneel and penetrate. The female can then arch her back. The male can then thrust.

1.

The female should start by sitting on the edge of a bed.

2.

Next, she needs to lie right back so that her head is on the bed. A pillow should be placed under her back to create an arch.

3.
The female should now shuffle forward slightly so that her bottom is now off the edge of the bed.

4.
The male should now kneel down on the floor facing her. He can now grab hold of the female's bottom and penetrate.

5.
The male can now thrust and should keep his hands on the female's bottom.

In this position, the male can hold on to the female's bum whilst having sex or a pillow can be used to support underneath it. The arch in the female's back is key to enhance the orgasm – it can be very easy to hit the G-spot by only making small changes in the position of the back.

Pretzel Dip
The female should lay on her side and have her partner straddle the leg that is on the bed. The other leg should wrap around his waist.

1.

The female should begin by lying down on her side on a bed.

2.

The female should raise her outer leg up into the air at this point while the male gets into position.

3.

The male should kneel down over the female's leg (the leg which is still on the bed).

4.

The male should then shuffle forward until close to the female's waist.

5.

The female should then wrap her leg (the leg in the air) around the front of the male's waist.

6.

The male should then grab the leg and lift it until he is able to penetrate.

7.

The male should keep hold of this leg as he begins thrusting.

G-Spot

The female should begin by lying on her stomach and then transitioning to face sideways in one direction. She can then bend her legs at the knee to support herself and keep balance. The male should approach her from behind on his knees for penetration. Once inserted, he may hold on to her waist while thrusting for harder and faster sex.

1.

The female should start getting into a sideways position. She can bend her legs for support and balance.

2.

Once in position, the male should kneel behind her and approach for penetration. It may help if the female opens her legs slightly for easier access.

3.

Once inserted, the female can close her legs and the male can hold on to her hips while he thrusts.

This one, obviously, is designed to hit the G-spot! So, keep that in mind! The male does all of the work in this position and it is designed for stimulating the female orgasm so enjoy!

This is also a great position when you want to start with one thing and end with another. For example, it's very easy to transition from this position to missionary or even doggy style during sex.

Slippery Nipple

The male should sit upright as the female lies flat on her back. She should place her legs either side of the male and inch forward. He can then do all the work during sex. The female can lie back and enjoy.

1.

The female should begin by lying down on her back facing the ceiling.

2.

The female should spread her legs wide and bend them at the knee with her feet flat against the bed.

3.

The male should kneel in front.

4.

The female should inch forward towards the male until he is able to penetrate her.

5.

Once inserted, the male has full control to lean back, but is able to lean right forward into a lowered missionary position and stimulate the nipples with his mouth hence the name.

The Clasp

The male should begin by standing up. The female can wrap herself around his waist and he can hold her up by placing his hands on her back and bum. Allow careful penetration and the female can raise herself up and down while the male carries her.

1.

This is a standing position and requires upper body strength. The male should begin by standing up. It may help for him to stand against a wall, to begin with.

2.

The female should approach him facing towards him.

3.

The female should wrap her arms around the male's shoulders and he should grab hold of her behind her back and under her bottom.

4.

Simultaneously, the female should lift off the ground and the male should help lift her up and above his waist.

5.

The male should then carefully lower the female on to his penis for penetration ensuring that he is still supporting her back and bottom.

6.

Once inserted, both the male and female should help intercourse by supporting the female moving in an up and downward thrust. If you are struggling with this position, it can be done against a wall rather than away from it. This way, the wall can support a significant portion of the female's weight and firmer thrusts can take place.

This is another position which can be done absolutely anywhere. It may require some upper body strength from the male – it can be quite hard to hold someone up for very long! It may be helpful if the female leans back against a wall or something else to support her during sex.

Reverse Cowgirl

This is a popular classic. The male should lay down flat on his back and the female should straddle on top of him, facing away instead of towards his face. The female can then move back and forth in complete control of the pace of sex.

1.

The male should lie down on a bed facing upwards. His legs should be slightly bent and slightly apart.

2.

The female should position herself over the male's waist and face away from him towards his feet.

3.

The female can kneel down with one leg on either side of the male's waist. She can then allow for penetration.

4.

Once inserted, the female can begin thrusting back and forth. The control from this is a great one for women and is often a popular position – some women find that they can't finish until they are on top and in control. The male benefits from having to do little work and gets a great view from behind. This can be quite a turn on.

Tight Squeeze

This is a position for adventurous sex and is best done somewhere other than the bedroom.

The female should sit down on somewhere and wrap her legs around her partner and 'tight squeeze'. The male should be standing, and the female's arms can wrap around him for support. This allows for close and intimate sex wherever you are.

1.

The female should find somewhere sturdy and secure to sit up on to such as a kitchen countertop or a table.

2.

The female should then shuffle close to the edge and open her legs. She may find it useful to position her hands behind her for support at this stage.

3.

The male can then approach from the front and position himself between her legs for penetration.

4.

Once inserted, the female should wrap her legs tightly around the male's body and squeeze, bringing him close.

5.

The female can now finally also wrap her arms around the male's neck and shoulders.

6.

Finally, although the male is in control during intercourse, the female is in a great position to influence the male's thrusts and movements as she pleases.

Lust and Thrust

The female should lay down on her back off the edge of the bed with her feet on the floor. She should raise her body and support herself on her arms with elbows bent. The partner should stand in front for penetration and lean down with his arms on either side of her body.

1.

The female should lie down on her back on a bed with her bottom and legs off the edge of the bed.

2.

The female should raise her body from the bottom down by positioning her elbows on the bed to support her and using her arms to help lift.

3.

The male should now position himself in front of the female and penetrate the female.

4.

Finally, the male should lean forward and position his arms either side of the female's body during intercourse.

5.

Alternatively, the male may remain standing and hold on to the female's waist while thrusting.

This position is great for getting close and intimate during sex without compromising thrust or pace. There is minimal work for the female to do during this position and both partners are well supported and secured.

Afternoon Delight

The female should lay on her side and slightly raise her outer leg to allow easier access. The male should penetrate from the side. Once inserted, the female can relax and lower her outer leg back down to the resting position.

1.

The female should begin by lying down on her side. It is best for her to maintain a slight bend in her legs at the knee.

2.

The female should slightly raise her outer leg to allow easier access for penetration. It may be useful for the female to use her hands to help support her leg whilst in the air.

3.

The male should approach from behind the female and shuffle into position for penetration.

4.

Once inserted, the female can relax her outer leg and lower is back to the resting position.

5.

The male is then free to thrust gently.

This is a good lazy position when you want to have sex, but don't have much energy!

Half on, Half off

The female should start by laying on a bed, legs off the end. The male can then stand and penetrate whilst the female wraps her legs around his.

1.

The female should begin by lying down on the edge of the bed. Her legs should be hanging off the edge.

2.

The female should open her legs outwards to allow access for the male.

3.

The male can now approach from the front and position himself for penetration.

4.

Once inserted, the female should lift her legs up and wrap them around the male's before having sex. If the bed is low, the male can kneel instead.

This is a good one for reaching the G-spot without having to do too much work!

The Ship

The male should lay down on his back. The female should then sit down on his penis and face sideways so that both of her legs are over on one side of his body.

1.

The male should begin by lying down in the basic position on a bed i.e. facing upwards, legs slightly bent and apart.

2.

The female should now position herself above the waist. However, she should face to the side of the male and both feet should be next to each other on only one side of the male.

3.

The female can down lower herself to allow for penetration.

4.

Both of the female's legs should now be on one side of the male's body. The female may now position her hands behind her on the opposite side of the male's body for support.

This is a position where the female is in control and can be good if she needs to be on top in order to finish.

y

The female should begin by lying face down on the bed. She should move closer to the edge so that her head and upper body hang off the bed towards to floor, using her hands for support. The male can then penetrate.

1.

The female should begin by lying face down on a bed.

2.

The female should now shuffle towards the edge of the bed and position herself so that her head and upper body completely hang off the edge. She may need to use her hands and arms to support her weight on the floor at this point.

3.
The male should now kneel now behind the female with the aim of penetrating from behind. This is best done from a kneeling position behind her with legs either side of the female.

4.
The male can now penetrate.

5.
The male should help support the female's body while she is hanging off the bed. This can be done by firmly holding on to the female's waist, or by having the male hold on to the female's hands and pulling them back. This is best for when things get rough!
Again, this position is designed for the ultimate orgasm with an increased blood flow to the head and all the effort being done by the male.

The Cat

The male lies down on top of the female in the missionary position. He then penetrates her as much as he can, bringing his body up against hers. Instead of thrusting, he can then move his hips in small circles to stimulate the clitoris with the bottom of his penis.

1.

The female should begin by lying down face up on a bed with her legs slightly bent and apart.

2.

The male should now position himself on top in the missionary position.

3.

The male can now penetrate.

4.

Once inserted, the male can push upwards into the female's body so that he is positioned slightly further up with the aim of causing more stimulation on the clitoris.

5.

Finally, instead of thrusting, the male should rotate his hips in a circular motion to cause more friction on the clitoris and increase stimulation.

This is great for women who need clitoral stimulation to orgasm. Just make sure both of you are comfortable in the position. It is very easy to switch between the standard missionary position and this position, so try mixing it up!

Closed for Business

This is an oral sex position. The female should lay down on her back with her legs 'closed for business'. The male can then go down on her.

1.

The female should lie down on her back and face upwards. Her legs should remain closed and together, but completely straight.

2.

Secondly, the female should raise her hips up in to the air and position her feet behind her head as shown in the illustration.

3.

The male can now kneel over her legs, facing her.

4.

The male can now lean forward and begin having oral sex with the female.

This position emphasises clitoral stimulation.

Happy Birthday!

The male should lie down on a bed with his feet on the floor. The female should get on top with her legs either side of him and guide his penis into her vagina.

1.

The male should lie down on a bed but ensure that his feet remain on the floor.

2.

The female should now position herself over the male's waist a face him.

3.

The female can now lower herself down to allow for penetration. Once inserted, it is best for the female to assume a kneeling position with one leg either side of the male's.

4.

The female can now begin thrusting back and forth or, if she leans forward towards the chest of the male, she can thrust up and down.

The best part about this is that the female is in overall control, but the male can use his legs to help thrust and get faster when reaching climax. He also gets a great view.

Organ Grinder

The female should lie on her back with her legs apart and raise them up into the air. The partner should kneel down and forward between her legs. He can then hold the legs up as he thrusts.

1.

The female should lie on her back with her legs apart and bent. The female should raise her legs up into the air. She may find it helpful to use her hands to support her legs up in this position until the male is in position.

2.

The male can now kneel in front of the female and move forward between her legs.

3.

The male can now penetrate the female.

4.

Once inserted, the male should hold on to the female's legs and keep them up in the air while he thrusts. By holding the thighs of the female, the male can use her legs to help him provide firmer thrusts.

This is a great one for reaching the G-spot and finishing sex.

The Mermaid

Find a surface that is flat and have the female lay down facing up with her bum at the edge. A pillow or something similar should be used to raise the hips safely and comfortably. The female should raise her legs up above and keep them closed. The male can then stand and penetrate – he can hold on to her legs to keep them secured.

1.

The female should find a flat surface such as a bed, kitchen countertop or table. A pillow can be used for comfort and support.

2.

The female should raise her legs right up into the air as a 90-degree angle to her body. She should keep them closed and keep her feet together. She may use her hand to support her legs in this position until the male is in position.

3.

The male can now approach from the front in a standing position and penetrate the female.

4.

The male should hold on to the legs and keep them in the air
and together.

5.

The female can now place her hands by her side for support.
Alternatively, she can place her elbows behind her and support
herself from this position.

Again, keeping the legs together will cause a greater sensation
for the male where there is more rubbing on the inside of the
vagina. The elevation is used to make it easier to hit the G-spot.

Pretzel

The female should lay on her side, have her partner straddle her
leg and bring the other leg around his waist. This gives good
penetration and the male will have his hands free for clitoral
stimulation or support if needed.

1.

The female should lie down on her side. Her legs should be
straight at this point.

2.

The male should kneel down over the lower leg and lift the
female's outer leg up while he approaches for penetration.

3.

This leg outer leg should now be wrapped around the front of the male's waist.

4.

The male can now penetrate.

5.

Once inserted, the male may use his hands for support or he may stimulate the clitoris.

Back Breaker

The female should lie on the bed with her legs hanging off the edge. She should shift her bum forward until it is also just off the edge. The male should kneel down in front of her and penetrate. The female can push up with her toes and arch her back. The male can then hold up her bum and thrust.

1.

The female should begin by lying down on a bed with her legs off the edge and her feet on the floor. She should be facing upwards.

2.

The male should approach from the front for penetration.

3.

Once inserted, the female should use her feet to push her body upwards and cause an arch in her back.

4.

When arched, the male should grab hold of the females bottom to help her maintain the position and begin thrusting. This position requires most effort to be done by the male, but having the female push with her toes and change the arch in her back can make it much easier to hit the G-spot.

The Bumper Car

This is a thrilling sex position which allows for deep penetration. This is great if you require G-spot stimulation to reach orgasm. Again, this position requires penile flexibility, so make sure the male is comfortable with the position.

Start with the female laying down on her stomach with her legs wide open and straight out. The male should then lie down on his stomach, with his legs open and straight out. He must be facing in the opposite direction. Afterwards, the male reverses back towards his partner so his thighs are resting over hers. He needs to do this until he is able to point his penis towards his partner's vagina. Then penetrate slowly.

1.

The female should lie down on her stomach facing downwards. Her legs should be open as wide as comfortably possible and straight.

2.
The male should position himself facing away from the female by her feet.

3.
The male should also lie down on his stomach, legs open wide and straight.

4.
Once in position, the male should slowly begin moving backwards so that his thighs rest over the female's.

5.
From this point, the male should focus on guiding his penis towards the vagina and penetrate slowly, ensuring that both partners are comfortable.

6.
Once inserted, the male can begin thrusting back and forth.
Safety Tips

This position requires penile flexibility. If you want to find out if the male's penis is flexible enough, have him stand against a wall. Pull his penis gradually down. If the penis is able to point directly down to the ground without causing pain then you should be fine to perform this position, but still be careful. The female should stay still when the male is initially penetrating her. The female should wait while he finds the most comfortable position and angle to thrust without injury.

Butter Churner

For this position, the female should lay on her back and bring her feet over her head so that the bum is up in the air. The male should stand over and squat up and down, coming completely out of the vagina each time.

1.

The female should lie down on her back.

2.

The female should bring her legs right up so that her bottom is in the air and bring her feet back over her head.

3.

The male should now stand in front of the female with his feet by her bottom.

4.

The male should now squat down for penetration.

5.

Once inserted, the male should continue squatting up and down, penetrating and re-penetrating the female each time.

This position will feel like the male is penetrating for the first time every time he penetrates which can be really satisfying.

Kneel and Sit

The male should kneel on a bed and the female should straddle him with her legs either side. The female has to control and choice in this position – sit, grind or move up and down. It's up to you!

1.

The male should begin by kneeling on a bed or anywhere else that seems comfortable.

2.

The female should approach the male from the front and straddle his lap with one leg on either side of the male. The female should be on her feet rather than on her knees and should be facing away from the male.

3.

The female can then position herself to allow for penetration.
The male has good access to the female's upper body in this
position.

Wraparound

The male should sit on a floor with his legs out. The female
should straddle and wrap her legs around him and carefully
allow him to penetrate her.

1.

The male should sit down on the floor with his legs out in front
of him.

2.

The female should position herself above the male, facing him
and with one foot either side of the male's legs.

3.

The female can now lower herself to allow for penetration.

4.

Once inserted, the female should wrap her legs around the back
of the male.

5.

For support, the male can either wrap his arms around the female or lean back on his arms.

This position is great as it gives some control back to the male. You are able to stay close and kiss whilst having sex without compromising the amount of penetration.

The Landslide

The female should begin by laying down looking at the floor. She should rest upon her forearms with her legs apart. The partner should sit behind and over her legs, also leaning back on his arms behind him. He should then penetrate and begin having sex.

1.

The female should start by lying face down on the floor.

2.

The female places her forearms below her chest and rest on them. Her legs should also be apart at this point.

3.

The male should then sit behind the female on his knees. His legs should be over hers and on both sides i.e. outside of her legs.

4.

The male can now position himself to allow for penetration.

5.

Once inserted, the male should lean back on his hands with his arms stretched out behind him.

By having the female close her legs, the male will feel fuller inside and it is much easier to find the G-spot.

Lap

This is a simple position. The male should sit up, using a wall or headboard to support him. The female sits on top and both can rock together.

1.

The male should sit up in front of a wall or a headboard with his legs crossed.

2.

The female can now position herself facing towards the male and above his lap.

3.

The female should now lower herself in a squat to allow for penetration. She can remain with her feet on the floor or on her knees.

4.

Once inserted, the female is in control and can rock back and forth.

This is a good position for a long sex session.

Home Fitness

In this position, both the male and female get into the push-up position. The female should be on the bottom and can use her knees to support. The male penetrates her from behind. This is a VERY exhausting position but can be worth the effort!

1.

The female should begin by getting into a press-up position. She may find it easier to rest on her knees.

2.

The male should position himself over the female in the press-up position.

3.

The male should carefully penetrate the female – he may use one of his arms to help penetrate if he has the strength to hold up his weight on one arm.

Shoulder Stand

The female should start by being on her back and the male should kneel in front. She should wrap her legs around and allow him to penetrate. He supports her with one hand on her back and she can then shift all her weight on to her shoulders. He can now thrust.

1.

The female should begin by lying down on her back with her legs open and slightly bent.

2.

The male should kneel in front of the female and move towards her to allow for penetration.

3.

Once inserted, the female should wrap her legs tightly around the male's back and bottom.

4.

The male should now place either one or both hands on the female's back to support her.

5.

The female can now lift her back until all of her weight is supported by her shoulders. She should maintain this arch position throughout intercourse.

The be secure and safe, the male should always provide support to the female.

This position allows for very deep penetration and incredible orgasms.

Dinner Time

The female should sit on a sofa on the edge. The partner should kneel in front and be between her legs. He can hold her thighs to get some more control as he engages in oral sex.

1.

The female should sit straight up on the edge of a sofa. Alternatively, she can lean back flat.

2.

The male should kneel in front of the female and take hold of her thighs.

3.

The male should spread the female's legs wide and engage in oral sex.

4.

The female should relax her legs so that the male has full control of their position throughout oral sex. If she resists or has impulses, the male should restrain her from moving – he is in control!

Face Sitter
This is an oral sex position – the name says it all here!
The male should lay down on his back. The female should lower herself above his face. Do NOT put all your weight down – the female should support herself using a wall or the bed. The female is in complete control of where his tongue is going.

1.
The male should lack down on his back.

2.
The female should position herself over the male's head facing either way.

3.
The female can now squat down until the male is able to begin oral sex.

4.
The female must remember to support all of her weight throughout this position. She is in total control of how the male's mouth is positioned and what it does.

The Thigh Master

This position is a variation of the cowgirl position. To begin with, the female should be on top facing away from the male. The male's knees should be raised to give the female something to support her.

1.

The male should lie down in his back with his legs apart and slightly bent.

2.

The female should position herself above his waist and face towards him.

3.

The female can now kneel down with one leg either side of the male to allow for penetration.

4.

Once inserted, the male should bend his legs further whilst keeping his feet firmly flat on the bed.

5.

The female should rest back against the male's bent legs as she uses her hips only to thrust back and forth.

Being on top is generally great for the female orgasm, but having the male's knees up will make his sensation better inside the female and you can both have a better orgasm together.

The Staircase

The female should sit on some stairs with her back leaning against one of the walls. The male should be standing a bit further down. The female should lift one leg up as the male penetrates her. He can then begin thrusting.

Just make sure no one else is around!

1.

Locate an appropriate staircase!

2.

Have the female sit on the staircase several steps up from the male. This will depend on the height of both partners so you may need to find what is most comfortable for you both.

3.

The female should lift one of her legs up on to the male's shoulders and rest them there throughout this position.

4.

The male can then penetrate, using the female's raised leg for support and to aid with firmer thrusts.

Kneeling Wheelbarrow

This one is easier than the one we tried earlier! The female starts off on all fours, putting her weight on to one forearm and one knee. The partner then kneels down behind and penetrates the vagina. This is another great one for hitting to G-spot.

1.

The female should start by getting down on her hands and knees.

2.

The female should then move on to her forearms instead of on her hands.

3.

The female should now rest all of her weight on to one of her forearms and one of her knees on the same side.

4.

The male should now kneel behind the female and penetrate, holding on to both of the female's upper legs when thrusting.

Dinner is Served

The female should wrap her legs around her partner and have him hold her bum in a carrying position. He should then penetrate. The female can then begin to lean back until parallel to the floor.

1.

The male should begin by standing in front of the female.

2.

The female should then, holding on to the male's shoulders, jump up and wrap her legs around the back of the male. Think of this as a carrying position.

3.

The female should then allow for penetration.

4.

Once inserted, the male should grab a firm hold of the female's hands and allow her to lean right back until her body is parallel to the floor.

5.

The female can now begin using her legs to help her thrust up and down.

This position is really fun and for both partners. It does require some upper body strength though! If this position is too difficult in terms of strength required, the female can rest her back on a bed instead of being elevated in the air parallel to the ground.

Ballet

This is an exhaustive position that requires flexibility, stamina and strength from both partners. Rather than a unique sex position, this is better thought of as an exciting way to begin having sex.

The female must begin by standing on a surface close to other structures that can be used for support such as a wall or cabinet. She should then lunge forward and lower herself, while the male does the same. He should inch closer in order to penetrate. Either party can now control the depth of penetration for the best orgasm.

1.

The female should begin by standing on a surface which is close to other firm surroundings such as walls or heavy/ fitted furniture.

2.

The male should be standing in front of her.

3.

Once in position, the male should ready himself to catch the female and support all of her body weight.

4.

The female should lunge forward towards the male. He should be ready to support her. It is best for the male to catch the female by holding her under the shoulders. When caught, she should be positioned around the male's shoulder area.

5.

The male can then lower the female while she keeps her legs out straight to the sides.

6.

Penetration can then take place.
Balance is key! Be sure to use surrounding supports in case!

Leg Up!

You should both begin by facing each other. The female should raise one leg up and wrap it around the male's leg, pulling him closer.

1.

Both the male and female should begin by standing and facing one another.

2.
The female should raise one leg up and bend it at the knee.

3.
The female should then use her leg and wrap it around the male's. She can then use her leg to bring him closer for penetration to take place.

4.
The female should keep her leg wrapped around the male for the entirety of this position.
This is great when you can't find a bedroom to have sex or just want to mix things up a bit!

Dirty Dancing
This is another anywhere, anytime move but the support of a sturdy object may be helpful when you haven't tried it before.

The male should lean on a wall facing the female and hold her. She should straddle him and wrap her legs around for balance.

1.
The male should lean back against a wall, facing the female.

2.

The female should hop up on to the male and wrap her legs around his back. He should use his hands to support her from the bottom.

3.

The female should now allow for penetration.

4.

Once inserted, the female can use the male's shoulders to help her move up and down during sex.

This is an intimate position where the male has a lot of access to the female's upper body. The penetration and clitoral stimulation can be controlled easily.

Leapfrog

Leapfrog is very much like the doggy style position that was covered earlier in this book – it is a variation of the doggy position.

For this position, you should start in the typical doggy style pose, but the female should lower her head and arms so that they are resting on the bed. The partner should then continue to penetrate from behind like usual.

1.

The female should begin by getting down on her hands and knees facing away from the male.

2.

The female should then lower her upper body by transitioning from resting on her hands to resting on her forearms. Her bottom should remain up in the air and she should arch her back inwards.

3.

The male should kneel behind the female, just like the doggy style, and approach for penetration.

4.

The male can then thrust firmly.

The great thing about this position is that penetration becomes much deeper than usual and it also frees up the hands. It is also great for getting a bit rougher than the normal doggy style positions.

69

This is perhaps one of the wider known and popular foreplay positions. For this, the male should lay down facing upwards. The female should straddle on top facing the male's feet end. She should stretch out on top of the male and begin oral sex, while he does the same.

1.

The male should begin by lying down on his back on a bed and face upwards. His legs should be slightly apart, but straight.

2.

The female should then position herself by kneeling over the stomach of the male with one leg either side. She should be facing away towards the male's feet.

3.

The female can then begin shuffling backwards until her waist is position above the male's face for oral sex.

4.

The male can then engage in oral sex.

5.

The female can now lean forward so that her face is above the male's waist. She can then also engage in oral sex at the same time as the male.
Both partners benefit from this position and can be great for stimulation before having sex.

The Hinge

The male should begin by kneeling upon a bed and leaning back to support his own weight. The female should face away, positioned in the doggy pose. She should lean down on to her forearms and move backwards until he has penetrated and begin having sex. This is good for keeping control of the penetration and speed.

1.

The male should begin by kneeling on a bed and leaning backwards. He should position his arms behind him to help support his weight in this position.

2.

The female should then face away from the male in front of him. She should get into the doggy style position i.e. on her hand and knees.

3.

The female should lean forward on to her forearms and raise her bottom.

4.

The female can now shuffle back towards the male to allow for penetration.

5.

Both the male and female can thrust up and down in this position.

The Missionary 180

This position puts a spin on the traditional missionary position, but it requires the male to be flexible!

First, the female needs to lay down on her back with her legs spread apart. The male then lies on top, but with his head down towards her feet – his legs should then be on either side of her body. Once in position, the male should carefully push his penis downwards and penetrate his partner. Get comfortable and perform upward and downward thrusts.

1.

The female should lie down on her back facing upwards.

2.

The male should then position himself on top of the female, but with his head towards her feet. The male should be using his arms to bear his weight at this point or, alternatively, be resting his weight on his elbows.

3.

The male must now position his legs either side of the female if not done so already.

4.
The male should now slowly lower his middle section and begin pushing his penis back and towards the vagina. The female may help guide the penis while the male supports his weight.

5.
Once inserted, the male can begin upward and downward thrusts.
Safety Tips

This position requires the male to have a very flexible penis – make sure he is comfortable before committing to the position! There is a risk of him straining his penis's suspensory ligaments. If he does feel any significant pain you should consider leaving the position behind and finding something better suited and comfortable. When entering the position, the female should be careful not to pull hard on the penis while guiding it inside her.

Conclusion

Thank you for making it through to the end of Kama Sutra Sex Positions. Let's hope it was informative and able to provide you with all of the tools you need to achieve your goals whatever they may be.

The next step is to share what you have learned with your partner, so that together you may try out all of the ancient secrets contained within the Kama Sutra. From the different ways to embrace all of the unique kisses, there are plenty of options contained within this book to truly help you begin each and every intimate moment. And once you are ready to begin getting intimate, there are numerous positions that are contained within this book just waiting for you to play around with.

You may have started out this book confused as to why such an ancient piece of literature is still held up today as one of the most well-known books on sexual intercourse, but we hope that after reading through you have discovered much of what the Kama Sutra has to offer. With such a rich and vibrant history, there is much more to the Kama Sutra than just some exotic positions, and instead, it details an entire way to live so that you can enjoy all the pleasures of life.

Too often we become absorbed in work, family life, and home our never-ending list of obligations and we forget that life is supposed to be enjoyed. We rarely hold pleasure up as one of the main goals in life, and it is time that we change our mindsets and embrace the fact that life has much more to offer us. No longer do you need to drudge through each day, only to wake up and begin the routine all over again. Instead, let this book be a lesson to you that pleasure is equally as important as duty, and to truly have a balanced life you must indulge in both.

Whether sexual or non-sexual, romantic, or non-romantic, there is so much pleasure within our world that we deprive ourselves of, or simply don't even know exists. The Kama Sutra reminds us to slow down and allow ourselves the freedom to explore our innermost wants and desires, so that we may see the true beauty in life. The Kama Sutra is spiritual in nature, and it doesn't matter if you believe in a religion or not, you too should be able to see the profoundness that is contained within. Allowing yourself to reach a higher plane of fulfillment is indescribable, and thankfully this book can help guide you to that place.

So, take a moment, close your eyes, and think about everything that makes you feel alive. Now, give yourself the freedom to partake in all of those pleasures, and then you will truly understand the power of the Kama Sutra.

Finally, if you found this book useful in any way, a review on Amazon is always appreciated!

Printed in Great Britain
by Amazon

21752741R00192